PARKINSON'S:
A Personal Story
of Acceptance
By
Sandi Gordon

BRANDEN PUBLISHING COMPANY
Boston, MA

Library of Congress Cataloging-in-Publication Data

Gordon, Sandi.
    Parkinson's : a personal story of acceptance / Sandi
        Gordon. p. cm.
    Includes bibliographical references and index.
    ISBN 0-8283-1949-9
    1. Gordon, Sandi--Health.
    2. Parkinsonism--Patients--United States--Biography.
I. Title
RC382.G67 1992
362.1'96833'0092--dc20   91-37486
[B]   CIP

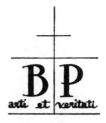

BRANDEN PUBLISHING COMPANY, Inc.
17 Station Street
Box 843 Brookline Village
Boston, MA 02147

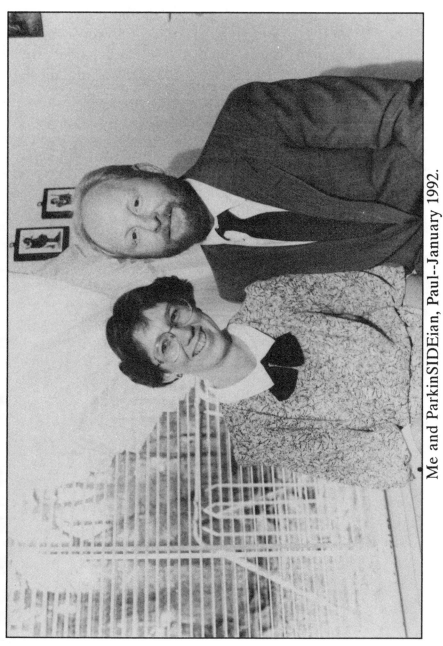

Me and ParkinSIDEian, Paul--January 1992.

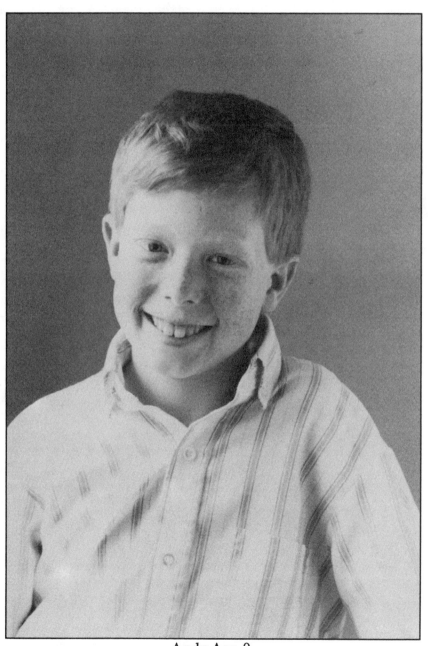

Andy-Age 9.

Dedicated:
to my loving and always supportive husband, Paul,
and
to my children, Andy, Becky, Stephanie and Gina.

Contents

FOREWORD 9
Chapter 1
    The Warning Signs 13
Chapter 2
    The Ultimatum 33
Chapter 3
    Some Good News 41
Chapter 4
    The Road to Acceptance 63
Chapter 5
    A Family Affair 79
Chapter 6
    A Laughing Matter 99
Chapter 7
    Setting Goals 109
Chapter 8
    The "ParkinSIDEian" 125
CONCLUSION 141
APPENDIX I 145
APPENDIX II 147
APPENDIX III 150
APPENDIX IV 151
APPENDIX V 153
NOTES 157
INDEX 158

FOREWORD

As a neurologist with a particular interest in Parkinson's disease and other movement disorders, I feel very honored to have been asked to write the foreword for this book. Sandi Gordon's well written and highly perceptive personal account speaks to everyone who faces situations of personal challenge--not just those with Parkinson's disease or their immediate families. I clearly remember the first day that Sandi Gordon and her husband, Paul, came to my office. She was 30 years of age--not many years younger than myself, and was forced to deal with Parkinson's disease, a progressive neurological disease that usually affects someone twice our age! There was no doubt about the diagnosis that day, and that her main problem at the time was the presence of unwanted, involuntary twitching and jerking movements (dyskinesias)--a side effect of the medication.

Since that time I have had nothing but increasing respect for this intelligent, intuitive, strong young woman. The way has not been easy. Whether young or old, it never is. Yet, for Sandi Gordon, it has been more difficult than usual. Unlike many Parkinsonians, she has not been robbed of graceful leisure in retirement years, nor has she had to go on disability rather than pursuing a promising career. Instead, she has had to somehow continue her full-time career as a mother of four young children. She has met the challenge by taking one day at a time rather than being overwhelmed by the situation, and giving up. Her success shows real strength, and makes her an important role model for others. Her husband, children, relatives and friends have likewise been strengthened by this growth experience.

Just as time has not stood still, neither has Sandi Gordon. During an office visit, she casually mentioned her disappointment that the local support groups were not relevant to a young adult with Parkinson's disease. I certainly empathized with her, knowing the many unique situations in which she found herself. However, it wasn't long before she had organized the first support group for younger Parkinsonians in the St. Louis area, and it was meeting in the Gordons' living room.

Then, another growth experience quickly loomed on the horizon. Seizing the opportunity, she went to the national convention of the American Parkinson Disease Association where she took part in a panel discussion to help spread the idea of support groups for younger Parkinsonians.

Eventually, it came as no surprise to me that she took on the challenge of writing this book--fueled by an intense desire for others to learn about Parkinson's disease, to learn from her personal experiences, and most importantly, to hear the underlying message of hope and the call to battle against the disease. A positive outlook and a determined drive are crucial-- this is really the crux of Sandi Gordon's book. Living with a chronic illness always involves loss, and the coping process takes time. However, a healthy mental attitude has tremendous value.

Another important message of Sandi Gordon's book is that effective management of Parkinson's disease requires a teamwork approach, which includes the patient, physician, therapists, family and friends. Long gone should be the days when patients went to the doctor and followed the doctor's orders without question. We now recognize how critically important it is for the patient to be an active participant in managing this chronic illness.

We have entered an exciting time of ever expanding knowledge about Parkinson's disease. Several new medications have recently been released and more will be on the way. There is much to hope for. Meanwhile, it will be largely due to the Sandi Gordons that the battles of Parkinsonians will be easier, and that eventually the war *will* be won.

Lee W. Tempel, M.D.
Movement Disorders Clinic
Washington Univ. Dept. of Neurology

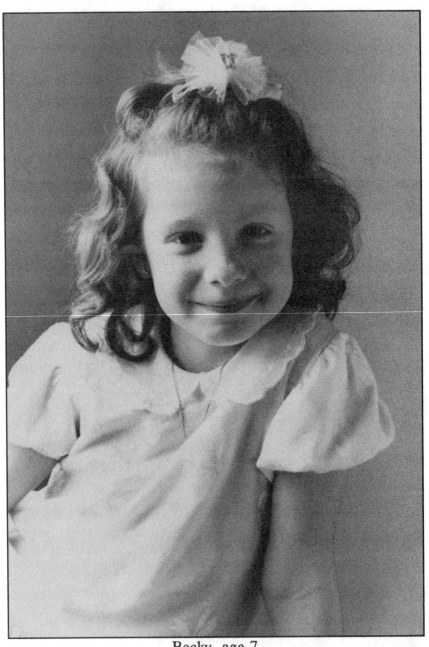

Becky--age 7.

Chapter 1
The Warning Signs

Prior to the summer of 1986, I perceived that my life was perfect. My thirtieth birthday was approaching, and there had never been a true crisis in my lifetime. I had grown up, sheltered from the injustices of life, in a loving and close-knit family, as the youngest of three children. We lived in a modest, middle-class home in a suburb of St. Louis, Missouri.

After accumulating more than my share of fond, carefree childhood memories, I was provided with the encouragement and financial means to venture away from home and attend college. Mastering both the skills to live independent of home, and to function on a mere three hours of sleep, I graduated with honors four years later from the University of Missouri in Columbia, earning a teaching degree in Special Education.

Marriage to my high school sweetheart, Paul Gordon, soon followed on July 28, 1979. Tracking the footprints of Good Fortune, I also landed my first teaching position that summer in a classroom of educable mentally handicapped youngsters. Upon acquiring three years of teaching experience to tack on to my resume, I was ready, and Paul was willing, to pursue my true ambition in life, and raise a family.

Parenting had always been my number one aspiration. Even though by many people's standards, child rearing may not be considered sufficiently challenging, prestigious, or rewarding, parenting was, and still is, my ultimate career choice. Thus, according to my criterion, I deemed myself a success by the spring of 1986, when I was 27 years old with a doting husband, three enviable red-headed children, a home of our own near both our families, a highly excitable and outgoing beagle, and a reliable Ford station wagon. My life was a nearly perfect match to the picture of adulthood I had imagined throughout my youth. I had no major complaints, and was very thankful to have not only been spared adversity, but disappointment as well.

Unfortunately, my story does not end with "...and we lived happily ever after", for my bubble burst in the summer of 1986. Our third child, Stephanie, had made her grand entrance into the world in February. I was breast feeding her, as had been my tradition with my other two children. At some obscure point within the first few months of nursing Stephanie, I noticed a very elusive tremor in my left hand. The quiver emerged whenever the baby was cradled in my right arm to nurse, and I used my free left hand to situate her to begin feeding. Lasting only seconds as I undid a blouse button or tucked a diaper under the baby's chin, the incipient trembling would vanish suddenly, and not reappear for sometimes several days. There was no rhyme or reason to these intrusions, no pattern whatsoever. The shaking would slyly time its visits so that each stay lasted long enough to arouse suspicion, but was spaced far enough apart from the next to dismiss any concern, and to question whether the tremor had indeed ever occurred.

15--Parkinson's

In the beginning, my mind was so preoccupied with the unceasing needs of the children, the subtle tremor was readily ignored. My days were inundated with caring for a newborn, a 13 month old and a 3 year old, as well as staying on top of the bottomless hamper of laundry, and the surplus of toys laying everywhere, with the exception of in closets or on shelves. My nights were consumed by doing whatever could not be accomplished during the day, EXCEPT sleeping. It was quite easy to overlook the seemingly innocuous shaking, nonchalantly attributing it to tension, fatigue, or perhaps, low blood sugar.

I honestly expected the tremor to resolve itself in time. Experience had proven that life would become more settled as Stephanie neared her first birthday, and spells of colic and middle-of-the-night feedings became obsolete. Once peace and order were restored, the unwelcomed quiver would surely subside. Procrastination also provided a better alternative to confronting the situation because I had never been crazy about seeing doctors, equating them solely with bad news.

By the fall, though, the tremor became impossible to disregard, as it was surfacing at other times, besides when I nursed Stephanie. The intrepid quiver was presenting itself--completely unannounced and always uninvited--when I poured a glass of milk, combed my hair, or turned a page of the newspaper. The shaking was, without doubt, getting worse, to the point where it was adversely affecting the fine motor coordination of my left hand, and slowing down my efficiency--something I desperately needed to run a household of five.

Facing up to the inescapable fact that the tremor was not going to disappear on its own, I reluctantly made an appointment to see an internist, Dr. Starne.

On that chilly, overcast December afternoon of my scheduled visit, I was feeling fairly anxious because of a strong, unrelenting intuition that something was seriously wrong. When I arrived at the office, the huge, windowless waiting area was packed with other silent, solemn faces. Rather than burying my worries in a magazine, I waited in mounting suspense, listening attentively to hear who would be next to be summoned through the door. Finally called to take the stand, a nurse escorted me to an examining room.

Upon recording my weight and blood pressure, the nurse departed, leaving me perched nervously on the end of the examining table. Moments later I was greeted by a young, attractive man who introduced himself as Dr. Starne. He was tall and slender, towering around 6'4". His warm, comforting smile and his charismatic personality quickly put me at ease. After I shared my personal observations concerning the tremor, the doctor led me through a series of informal tests that required me to push, pull and squeeze in order to compare the strength of each of my hands. Then Dr. Starne scrounged around the room for various paraphernalia--a dull and a sharp stick, a tissue, a cotton ball and a pin--to use to assess my left hand's sense of touch. With my eyes closed, I was instructed to report each poke, prick, tickle and touch of my hand. The doctor concluded that my hand was still strong and had feeling, but the shaking was indisputable whenever I rotated my wrist back and forth. Dr. Starne's first impulse was to send me to a neurologist (which, as it turned out, would have been the wisest decision). However, after briefly discussing the problem with another colleague in the office, he opted instead to schedule me for a nerve conduction study on my left arm at a local hospital. The first available appointment was not until December 28. Unfortunately the fear and worry over the mysterious tremor, and the upcoming test, ruined my Christmas that year. Rather than cherishing this magical season with my children, I allowed their expectant looks and their delighted squeals to go unnoticed. Oblivious to my surroundings, I numbly stumbled through all the Christmas-time rituals-- assembling the advent wreath, baking the countless trays of tasty cookies, and hanging the sixty foot paper chain around the living room which our son, Andy, had proudly made when he was four years old. Nothing seemed to spark my emotions that Christmas.

I felt only depressed and cheated as I listened to jubilant carols singing of "comfort and joy," or opened presumptuous greeting cards wishing us a "merry" Christmas and a "happy" new year. The entire world seemed to be immersed in the fervor of the holiday festivities, bubbling with excitement and immune to sorrow. Meanwhile, I was mesmerized by visions of myself with some terminal illness, and tortured myself with the inexorable thought that this could possibly be my last Christmas.

The nerve conduction study was not a pleasant experience, but at least it didn't take long. The technician got right down to the task at hand, not wasting any time with idle chitchat in an effort to disarm my fears. It was just as well, though, for I was feeling quiet and unsociable--my only interest being to get through this test and away from the anguish associated with hospitals.

During the test, the technician strategically positioned pairs of electrodes in various spots on my arm. Then, electrical impulses were induced, which were not exactly painful, but were definitely discomforting. Because of the lack of communication prior to starting the procedure, I was alarmed and somewhat embarrassed at seeing my arm flinch nervously beside me, and having no means of controlling it. After each jolting electrical shock, a machine recorded the speed of the nerve carrying the impulse from the first electrode to the second one. The readings were later compared with a table of norms to check for a possible blocked or injured nerve.

After I paced for several agonizing days, Dr. Starne telephoned me with the results. My normal readings on the nerve conduction study ruled out complications with the motor component of the nerves in my arm, and thus, a host of serious problems. Great news! By process of elimination, the doctor deduced that there must be damage to the sensory component of a nerve in my arm, causing the tremor. Although I could distinguish between hot and cold or dull and sharp, and the difficulties with my hand were entirely related to movement, Dr. Starne elucidated that injury to the sensory part of a nerve can also adversely affect its motor ability, even if the motor part was not impaired. He advised me to simply allow it time to heal and to take supplemental vitamin B6, a nerve stimulant, to speed recovery. Upon hanging up the phone, I tried to breathe a sigh of relief, but couldn't. My original nagging premonition that something was terribly amiss still prevailed. Despite Dr. Starne's confident summation that time was the miracle panacea for my problem, I could not help but question the many discrepancies in his diagnosis. If there was sensory nerve damage in my arm, why could I readily differentiate all sensations in my hand? And, secondly, how had the nerve been injured? Perhaps the circulation in my arm had become obstructed during one of those many cozy occasions when Stephanie had fallen asleep nursing, curled up against my left arm for long stretches. Maybe I had slept too soundly and too long on my arm one night. Or possibly the nerve had been impaired when the IV needle was inserted in my arm during the baby's delivery. I groped for any explanations that would make sense out of Dr. Starne's theory, wishing to justify his diagnosis, and to believe everything would be fine if given sufficient time. His prognosis was far better than any I had envisioned! His verdict was replete with hope! So, in spite of my skepticism, I tried my best to push aside my overbearing concerns, redirecting my attention back on my family.

In the weeks that followed, however, my fears and doubts prevailed, having gained credibility. In addition to the tremor, other frightening symptoms were cropping up. I was losing my balance and frequently stumbling into walls and door frames, bruising elbows and shoulders. It was even difficult for me to maintain my balance when I was standing idly with both feet planted firmly on the floor. For no apparent reason, I would suddenly feel my body teetering over. Fortunately, instinct would then intervene, and send me scrambling forward or backward in an effort to regain my balance and prevent a fall.

I also began walking with a limp, dragging my left foot along. My quick, long-legged strides were replaced with short, shuffled steps. My arms no longer swung synchronously with every step, but were glued stationary to my sides. I had acquired a stooped posture as my shoulders slumped forward and my head hung down parallel with the ground.

My neck also seemed stiff. Whereas most people turn only their head to look to the side, I rigidly twisted my entire upper body. Nodding or shaking my head, especially, took deliberate effort. I often had to resort to a verbal "yes" or "no" on those many occasions when my head stubbornly refused to budge and someone was staring expectantly at me, waiting for my response to a query.

Communication was an odious chore. Writing had become tedious, and my handwriting was rapidly shrinking in size. What once earned an A+ in Penmanship, now appeared to be only scribbles and lines.

21--Parkinson's

My voice had become barely audible, and my speech was often slurred. Paul was constantly nagging me to "speak up." By the third or fourth time of asking me to repeat something I had said, he would glare at me impatiently and sharply demand, "What?!" in exasperation. This was confusing, because from my perspective, it seemed as though my voice was being projected normally. I could hear me just fine!

I was also experiencing strange sensations that would come and go mysteriously, such as a tingling "pins and needles" feeling up my spine, or an eerie, hot burning sensation in my leg. Sometimes, one of my hands would feel warm while the other hand oddly felt ice cold.

The most annoying symptom of Parkinson's was an awareness that my overall movements were abnormally laggard, as if my body were moving in slow motion. My mind was racing ahead full speed, but my hands could not move faster than a slow idle. (Later, I learned the medical term for this slowness is "bradykinesia.") Every task that I undertook demanded my full attention, as well as an exorbitant amount of time and perseverance, for I had to mentally command my uncooperative hands through each minuscule step along the way. Rather than flowing together as one swift smooth action, a skill as basic as slipping on a pull-over shirt ended up being quite an ordeal after it was broken down into its twelve separate steps, each one requiring serious contemplation to navigate. I plodded along with such slow and deliberate moves, I resembled a mechanical robot. It seemed as though it took forever to do even the simplest chores. To make matters worse, a baby, a two-year-old and a 4-year-old are not generally noted for their abounding patience. Their interminable demands and my inefficiency created a lot of frustration for everyone.

Paul first commented about my sluggishness one spring afternoon when we were changing the sheets on our bed. He watched as I very slowly and painstakingly inched my way down the side of the mattress, expending a great deal of effort and concentration to accomplish the onerous job of tucking in the sheets. Paul finally observed critically, "You never do anything fast anymore. It seems like you just can't hurry!"

Quite the opposite problem was a phenomenon later to be identified as "festination." Festination refers to a tendency to walk in very short, quick steps. The best analogy for this mannerism would be the descent of a precipitous hill. Despite your intentions to edge down the steep incline slowly and cautiously, you soon lose control and begin speeding heedlessly down the hillside, unable to stop.

It was most embarrassing to be walking through a crowded area when this problem chose to surface. I would suddenly find myself unable to brake in time to avoid bumping shoulders, or abruptly cutting off another person who happened to be innocently approaching a doorway at the same time. Poor Paul was my most frequent victim--and right in his own home!

I felt like a prisoner in my own body. Although I still had authority over my mind, I was quickly losing power over my actions--from walking to talking. As each new problem evolved, my fears were intensified. Fright had a way of aggravating my symptoms in such a way that, at times, it practically immobilized me. I could be effortlessly fixing dinner when one of my many unwelcome symptoms would unexpectedly leap forth, and divert my attention. As an inner alarm sounded, calling all worries, my outer faculties simultaneously shut down. In a split second, my body was stiff and rigid, and it took twice the effort to move at half the speed.

As a defense mechanism against the fear, I began denying the reality of the situation to myself and others. I naively attributed the various difficulties to the "sensory nerve damage" in my arm, expecting this to account for everything. This feeble excuse was also used to request help with chores that were a struggle for me--cutting my meat, wrapping a gift, or buttoning a shirt.

I was determined to believe my left hand would improve in time, and the other symptoms would dissipate into thin air. I rationalized that many of the newer problems were a result of my exorbitant anxiety over my hand, and that they would disappear once my nerve healed and I could once again relax. My theory was reinforced by the fact that my symptoms did indeed become more pronounced under stress.

Believing in mind over matter, I would wake up many mornings, decisively turning over a new leaf, and giving myself a pep talk in an effort to psyche myself up to act "normal" for the day. When my peculiar mannerisms failed to remain concealed, I was unfairly hard on myself--hating myself at times, and accepting full responsibility for my actions.

Feeling totally powerless as my physical condition deteriorated, I began relying more on my faith. All my personal attempts to intervene in my saga had been of no avail. Perhaps the Almighty God, the God of mercy, the God of miracles, the God who promised that we need only ask to receive, would rescue me from this plight. Striving for a closer relationship with Him, I became more active in our church by joining the handbell choir and teaching children's Sunday school.

Participating in the handbell choir only added to my already lengthy list of frustrating experiences, as I often unsuccessfully coordinated the necessary wrist action to sound the bell with the proper timing of the notes in the music. Teaching first grade Sunday school went no more smoothly with its repetoire of fine motor tasks--coloring, cutting, stapling and pasting. Even reading aloud a Bible story or conversing with the children vacillated on the edge of my capabilities.

I also started reading the Bible daily, and praying incessantly, earnestly pleading with God that my troubles not be the result of a terminal illness. Despite my outward attempts to deny the seriousness of the situation, I knew deep down that there was more to my problem than a damaged nerve. I worried about the possibility of a brain tumor.

Paul and I were bickering more than usual. Having not yet identified the true villain, Paul errone-ously targeted his anger at me--anger which was generally provoked by some trivial and irrelevant incident. Meanwhile, I was gradually becoming very dependent on him, physically and emotionally. Paul was regularly being solicited to help cook dinner, fold laundry, dress children, and wash dishes. What I yearned for most during this time of ineffable fear and uncertainty, though, were his compassion and his reassuring comfort. However, the closer I grew toward him, the farther he drew away from me. Paul felt utterly helpless as he witnessed each change overcome me, and frustrated at my refusal to face reality and seek a second doctor's opinion.

In the summer of 1987, Paul intimated that my condition might improve with more exercise. Wishing to please him and keep peace between us, I enrolled in an eight week class of aerobics. Anyone familiar with aerobics knows that it entails moving in a quick dance-like fashion, and thus, requires speed, agility, and coordination--all the skills I was lacking. Unable to keep pace with the other participants, it was a very humiliating experience. Although typically an outgoing person, I felt extremely self-conscious, and became quite introverted throughout the two months, never initiating conversation with anyone in an effort to gain a friend. Even though Paul was adamant that the aerobics class had noticeably improved my physical condition, I had no intention of putting myself through another eight weeks of embarrassment.

My next game plan was to concentrate on strengthening my left hand, which I believed to be the crux of my problems. After all, the quiver had been my earliest sign of trouble. Maybe by eradicating this instigator, the other symptoms would follow suit. At my request, my sister-in-law, an occupational therapist, demonstrated half a dozen exercises, using a hammer as a weight, to tone up my hand. After several weeks of doing the exercises faithfully, I became discouraged and quit. My arm and wrist were definitely stronger, but my hand shook as much as before.

That fall, we arranged a four-day visit with Paul's brother and his family in Douglas, Kansas. As we drove the 450-mile trek across the redundant expanse of Kansas, I was both relieved and hopeful....relieved to be escaping the drudgeries of home--the cooking, cleaning and laundry--and hopeful that this trip would be the turning point in a previously strained relationship with my sister-in-law, Beth.

The week-end started out following the usual pattern. The children were playing beautifully with their cousins, delighted at the opportunity to be together. Paul and his brother were chattering incessantly on their favorite topics--work, cars and airplanes. And Beth and I were being cordial but distant toward one another.

It was on the third day that an indiscreet remark by Beth retracted all hope for my dream of a reconciliation with her during this visit. That afternoon, when I was out of earshot, Beth approached Paul and asked point blank, "What's wrong with Sandi? She moves like an old lady." Respecting how sensitive the subject had become for me, Paul evaded the question. Later that evening, as Paul and I were chatting in bed alone, he shared Beth's terse observation, probably in an attempt to draw me out of my state of denial. In light of the existing animosity between Beth and me, I instinctively took offense. Feeling hurt and angry, I hurriedly packed our belongings the following morning so we could make our departure as early as possible. Once again, I had to flee from reality.

The trip did provide me with the needed incentive to return to Dr. Starne. A year had elapsed since my last appointment--ample time for the nerve to heal. After reexamining my hand, the doctor was favorably impressed by the increased muscle tone of my left palm, which was undoubtedly the result of the two months of hammer exercises. Noticing how upset and edgy I was, he calmly reassured me, recommended some additional exercises for my hand, and exhorted me to relax. How could I relax when I was convinced I was dying! But rather than risk having Dr. Starne confirm my fear, I timidly left the office without divulging the most recent symptoms.

Following the office visit, I was terribly depressed. It had become nearly impossible to laugh or even smile. I had to force myself out of bed every morning, dreading the start of each new day. In order to cope physically, I relied on others, especially my five year old son, Andy. I had learned to avoid calling upon Paul for help as he was quickly losing patience with me.

Although Andy is the mirror image of his father with his slate blue eyes, his strawberry blond hair, and the countless freckles sprinkled across his cheeks, I like to take, at least, partial credit for his good-natured disposition. Andy has always been a thoughtful and very outgoing person, never at a loss for friends. He has always amazed us at his ability to strike up a friendship instantly, while waiting at the pediatrician's office, swimming at the beach, or standing in line at the grocery store. His compassion for others is evident within our home, too. Andy is the peacemaker in our family, willing to sacrifice his last piece of Halloween candy, volunteer to take his turn last in a game, or give up the prize window seat in the van to appease his sisters.

Andy's generosity shone through during this tumultuous time in my life. He eagerly and willingly offered his help. I often enlisted him to put on and tie Stephanie's shoes, or to mass produce peanut butter and jelly sandwiches for lunch. Andy played a vital role in pulling me through the struggles of daily living. He became my right-hand man. His only motivator was, and still is, the personal reward he feels from pleasing others.

Since each chore took me two or three times longer to complete than the average person, I sought every measure imaginable to hoard time. Time was a precious commodity. Every nonessential task was eliminated in order to simplify my life, and to add a few treasured minutes to my days. Among the solutions employed, I frequently slept in my clothes, favored outfits without buttons or ties, and switched from contact lenses to glasses. Despite my fifteen years invested in wearing contacts, it had been costing me as much as an hour of my time to get them in or out.

The housework was neglected as well. Ironically, I had once been a very meticulous, organized person. In our early years of marriage, Paul had ribbed me because of my inability to leave home in the morning unless every bed was neatly made, or to go to sleep at night until every dirty dish was washed, dried and put away in its designated place. My previously immaculate home now, eight years later, had a wall-to-wall carpet of toys and children's dirty socks. Beds were rarely made, and clutter piled on the counters and table. Everything--dressing, cleaning, cooking, caring for the kids, eating, even talking--was a tremendous chore for me. I did only what was necessary to survive.

Our social life was naturally affected, as I sequestered myself within the confines of my own home. Friends and family were regularly cornering Paul to inquire about my health. Rather than risk an explosive confrontation with Paul over their concerned remarks, I began avoiding people whenever it was feasible. When we did entertain, all my energy was expended trying to disguise my problems. I had it down pat--the trick of serving finger foods to eliminate the aggravation of utensils, and of disappearing to the bathroom or kitchen "coincidentally" when it was my turn to shuffle and deal the cards.

Only casual acquaintances or strangers were directly confronting me--the pediatrician, the postal worker, people from church. It seemed every time I left home, someone would comment on my tiny handwriting, inquire about my limp, or compliment me on my extraordinary calm and patient temperament when

I interacted with my three energetic and, at times, rambunctious children. Little did they realize, my "patience" was actually the result of my having neither the strength nor the ambition to raise my voice. Each of these episodes out in public reinforced my feeling that the world was ganging up on me. I wished people would just leave me alone and stop caring!

At the end of January 1988, I finally resolved to return to Dr. Starne and confess everything--my stiff neck, my poor balance, my lopsided gait, and my overall slowness and lack of coordination. I even compiled a written list of my symptoms to be certain none were omitted. My depression and my quiet voice were not included for it did not seem viable to me that these traits could be related to my physical problems. However, my mood and subdued voice should not have eluded the doctor.

Throughout the examination, I was trembling uncontrollably and on the brink of tears. I was certain that, upon reading my list, Dr. Starne would react out of sheer panic, and point me directly to the hospital, without passing "GO," to confirm his suspicions (and mine, too!) of a possibly fatal brain tumor. Instead he glanced briefly at my scribbled notes. Seemingly unimpressed, he ordered me to walk up and down the endless corridor several times while he studied my gait. Then he called a nurse to draw my blood to check my thyroid level. Finally Dr. Starne prescribed the tranquilizer, Xanax, for what he believed were "stress-related" symptoms. He instructed me to telephone the office in a few days for the findings of the blood test, and again in two weeks to report on the success of the Xanax.

I went home, relieved that my problems did not constitute a serious illness, but also embarrassed at my inability to handle stress better. I felt like the little boy in the classic Aesop's fable, who repeatedly and groundlessly hollered "Wolf!"

After receiving confirmation that my thyroid was not the culprit, I impatiently waited the full two weeks, only to decide that there had been no visible change accredited to the medication. Feeling too humiliated by all that had transpired in the previous year and a half, I ceased taking the Xanax, but never called Dr. Starne.

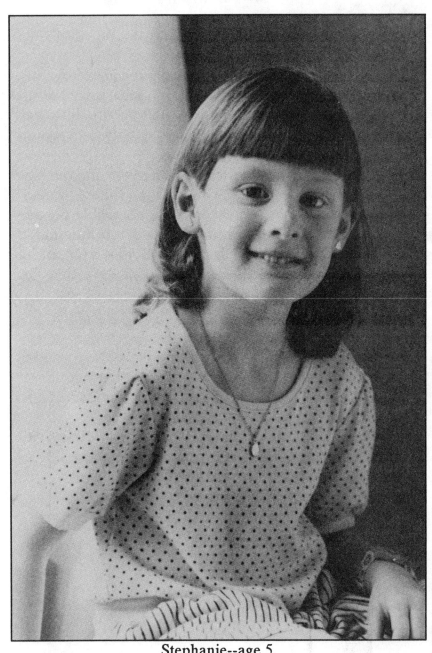
Stephanie--age 5.

Chapter 2

The Ultimatum

In February of 1988, Paul and I were shocked to discover I was pregnant. Number four would be arriving in late September. The news invoked very mixed emotions. Part of me was rightfully petrified at the thought of caring for a tiny, defenseless infant. I was already frantically struggling to keep up with the overwhelming demands of my current family. Another part of me was overjoyed, because of my love for children and parenting. Plus, because of my lifelong slender build, the extra pounds during past pregnancies had always been complimentary on me, particularly in my face. With the additional weight, the healthful diet, the extra rest, and the prenatal vitamins, pregnancy had always agreed with me. Thus, I hoped this fourth pregnancy would help me to magically snap out of my problems.

Surprisingly, Paul accepted the news very well. Throughout our marriage, he has always focused his thoughts on the present, rather than the past or the future. Paul's philosophy is that the past is over and done, and the future will care for itself. Instead of dwelling on what went wrong with our family planning, or how we were going to fit another child into our lives, Paul concentrated on the here and now. And the undeniable fact was, we were expecting another baby!

Our friends and relatives, on the other hand, were understandably concerned rather than excited for us. This was apparent from their awkward hesitancy when offering the traditional "congratulations". Their unspoken thoughts of "Oh, dear! How terrible!" were acutely amplified through their troubled, constrained silence. My only memory of anyone reacting with sincere happiness, was when we shared the announcement with Paul's mother. She was immediately overcome with the delightful prospect of another grandchild. (She undoubtedly must be the one responsible for shaping Paul's attitude toward living life in the present!)

Needless to say, there was no dramatic improvement during my pregnancy as I had naively hoped. Instead, the added stress of thirty pounds of extra weight, and of preparing the house and our lives for yet another little one, only magnified my symptoms. As the end of my pregnancy drew nearer, I became obsessed with worry. I doubted my ability to handle the awesome responsibility of caring for a helpless newborn. My hands were so slow and clumsy. It took me five minutes to fasten ONE button, eight minutes to peel and slice ONE carrot, and ten minutes to scrub ONE child's head of hair! How was I going to keep a demanding and impulsive infant fed, clean, dry and happy?

One muggy July evening, after still another worried family member had drawn Paul aside to share his concerns about me, followed by yet another tearful argument between Paul and I, Paul declared he had an ultimatum for me. Immediately my mind crowded with thoughts of separation and divorce. Paul had always been a very loving, devoted husband, and totally committed to the institution of marriage. However, judging by his stern, brusque tone of voice and the tense, irritated look on his face, it was obvious that Paul's thinning patience had finally worn through. I shuddered at the thought of receiving the dreaded judgement.

Paul gave me an icy stare as he curtly delivered the terms. He stipulated that either I make an appointment within two days to see a second doctor, or else he would schedule one for me. Feeling trapped, I tried desperately to squirm out of the situation, pleading with Paul to allow me to wait until after the baby came. I was sure that Paul was being unreasonably unfair, but he stood his ground firmly. He had reached his limit, and wasn't about to revoke his decision. So, for two days I anxiously debated whether to see another internist, a therapist, a psychiatrist, or a neurologist. Upon reaching my deadline, I reluctantly made a July 29 appointment with an internist named Dr. Simms.

On the eve of my check-up, Paul and I had arranged for a sitter to watch the children while we went out to dinner in honor of our ninth wedding anniversary. Although conversation was strained and trite throughout our meal, I was able to discern traces of Paul's steadfast love for me, as well as compassion for my fears. Despite my anger and resentment at Paul for forcing me to face my problems, I also harbored conflicting feelings of respect and admiration for Paul. He had not taken the easy way out, and given up on me and our relationship. His ultimatum was presented out of pure love. I was also thankful....thankful that Paul had taken the first step that I couldn't. I, too, needed answers.

The following afternoon, I shambled into Dr. Simms' office, eight months pregnant, and armed with another written list of my symptoms--only this time it was complete. Once introductions were completed, Dr. Simms listened sympathetically to my complaints, intent on catching every soft and mumbled word. He then guided me through a series of tests--many of which I have repeated innumerable times since that day. After observing my performance on such feats as walking a straight line, tapping my thumb with each successive finger as rapidly as possible, and, beginning with both arms straight out, touching my finger to my nose quickly and repeatedly, Dr. Simms referred me to a neurologist. It is my guess that he knew that day what was at the root of my troubles, but wanted the confirming opinion of a professional in the field of neurology. Paul and I were finally going to get some answers. I earnestly prayed for the courage to handle those answers!

The earliest date available to see the recommended neurologist was August 24, three days after my 30th birthday. Despite Paul's sincere and thoughtful offer to accompany me to the doctor's, I chose to go alone. It was my feeling that I would draw more inner strength to handle the verdict if Paul was not present to lean on emotionally. I sensed it would take all the strength I could muster to make it through that dreaded morning. Although it should have been the least of my concerns, and it would have been perfectly acceptable, I was overly concerned about crying in the presence of the doctor. Even though it was still mid-morning when I drove to the medical building, the temperature was already climbing near 90 degrees. It was going to be another scorching August day in St. Louis. When I entered the tiny waiting area, the room was very scantily furnished, and there was not a person in sight. Upon notifying the receptionist of my arrival, I slumped down into the nearest chair. Being a fan of impressionism, the soft, shimmering colors of a picture of the French countryside, painted by Claude Monet, distracted my worrisome thoughts.

Dr. Hastings, himself, greeted me in the waiting room, and led me back to his office. He was a short, gentle, white-haired man in his mid-60's. Much of the visit duplicated previous examinations, as the doctor checked my reflexes, posture, balance, gait, agility and coordination. Dr. Hastings was wearing a hearing aide, and had to strain to hear my faint, nervous voice throughout the neurological exam. This only reinforced his diagnosis--Parkinson's disease.

Parkinson's disease. While the name was familiar, my knowledge of this neurological disorder was extremely limited. I recalled that my 94-year-old Uncle Guy was said to have Parkinson's; how it affected him, I did not know. I had always erroneously attributed all his peculiar mannerisms to "old age". The impaling words, "Parkinson's disease", though, had an ominous ring to them, and instantly conjured up frightening thoughts. I anxiously pressed the doctor for a prognosis. I longed for a concise picture of my future, to know exactly what lay ahead. Realizing today the erratic course of Parkinson's from one individual to another, I can now appreciate Dr. Hastings' evasive responses to my anxious questions. Many of my worries had to remain unresolved.

Dr. Hastings explained that Parkinson's disease, for some unknown reason, causes death of certain nerve cells located in a part of the brain, the substantia nigra. These cells play a key role by producing the chemical dopamine. A lack of dopamine affects another area of the brain, the basal ganglia, which controls movement, and can cause stiffness, tremors, slowness, loss of balance, changes in gait, stooped posture, soft and slurred speech, and depression, among other symptoms. A hand tremor is typically, but not always, the first symptom. I fit the description to a tee, except for one thing--age. I was 30 years old with a disease that primarily strikes people in their 60's, 70's and 80's.

Dr. Hastings finished by saying, "The good news is the disease can initially be treated effectively with medicines. But the bad news is the disease is slowly progressive and has no cure." Diagnosis is based on observation, ruling out other possibilities and experimentation with antiparkinson drugs to determine if they will affect the symptoms. The doctor, therefore, ordered a blood test to rule out Wilson's disease, and an MRI brain scan to check for a tumor during my upcoming hospital stay to have the baby. Lastly, Dr. Hastings prescribed Sinemet, a powerful medication used in the treatment of Parkinson's.

I dejectedly headed straight to my car and drove to a deserted corner of the parking lot for a good cry. I desperately needed some quiet and prayerful time alone to sort out this devastating news. Paul and I had sensed something was seriously wrong, but had banked on the hope that the problem could be corrected, and then everything would be wonderful once again.

Upon sharing the crushing news with Paul that evening, we felt both distraught and relieved. At least we had finally reached the end of a two-year nightmare. There would be no more fear of the unknown, and no more second guessing. We now knew what we were up against. Paul and I felt a special closeness that night which had been absent for most of those prior two years.

Once again, Paul managed to put the past behind, refused to fret about the future, and instead, wisely focused on our present lives. Paul has always had an admirable ability to remain genuinely optimistic and confident during adverse times. This time was no exception. Paul was certain we would grow to accept our dubious challenge if we dealt with it just one day at a time.

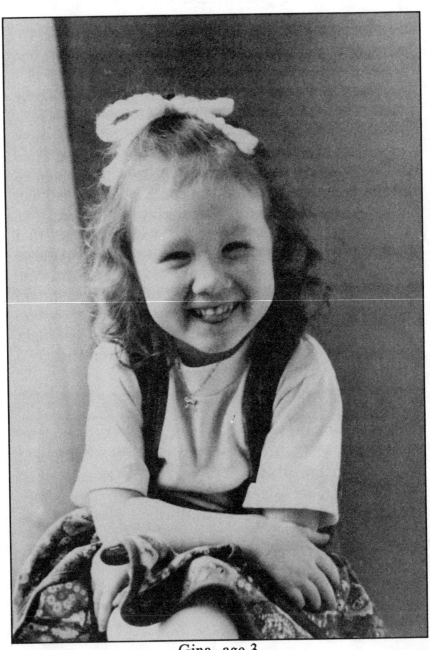

Gina--age 3.

Chapter 3
Some Good News

My diagnosis came just one month prior to the baby's arrival date. Dr. Hastings warned that it may take three or more weeks before noticing any effects from the Sinemet, and suggested we not delay starting this antiparkinson drug. By initiating drug treatment during my final month of pregnancy, there would be ample time to introduce the drug slowly into my system, thereby avoiding or, at least, minimizing nausea, a common side effect. Dr. Hastings planned to gradually increase my daily dosage, over the course of the month, to three tablets of Sinemet 25/100, in hopes of realizing some improvement in my symptoms before the delivery of the baby. After gaining approval from my obstetrician, I started taking the Sinemet, anxiously watching each day for any desired changes.

Changes snuck in so gradually and were so minute that, at the end of the three weeks, Paul and I weren't convinced that the Sinemet had produced any benefits at all. Yet, our friends and family remarked that they could see a subtle difference. I was still disappointed, having hoped for a 180 degree turn around--a new me. Later, I learned that stress dramatically influences the symptoms of Parkinson's disease. The ninth month of pregnancy was, therefore, not an optimal time to evaluate the effectiveness of the medications for controlling symptoms.

Paul and I spent what little time we had before our newcomer's scheduled appearance, accumulating as much information on Parkinson's disease as we could. I have never felt there was much truth in the old adage that claims "Ignorance is bliss." We had dozens of questions needing answers, and knew our reading time was about to be markedly reduced for several months with a new infant in the house.

We also began the painful job of breaking the depressing news of my diagnosis to friends and relatives. No longer feeling personally responsible for all the strange behaviors I had exhibited, it was now possible for me to objectively visualize myself as I had been over the last couple of years. Seeing myself from the eyes of those around me, prompted me to relay the facts. Everyone deserved an explanation for the alarming changes that had taken place in me. I generally confided the news in a letter or via the telephone. It was easier to share if I was not face to face with the other person. The distressing task inevitably generated tears, making it that much more difficult for both parties.

My obstetrician had scheduled me for a Caesarean section on September 23. The anticipation of the baby had been our source of power to help us surge forward through these rough times. It provided us with something hopeful on which to focus our attention. The responsibility of caring for a newborn challenged us to be strong, and was our motivator not to succumb to defeat.

43--Parkinson's

After ironing out every last detail of the childcare arrangements, from bus schedules to lunch money, we were ready for the big day, or so we thought. On that cool damp fall morning, the alarm sounded at 5:30, reminding us that we had only an hour before we were expected to report to the hospital. As we hurried out the door, Paul made the aggravating discovery that the camera batteries were dead. Thus began the hour long scavenger hunt across a sleeping town, in search of an open store that carried the correct replacements. Finally succeeding at our mission, we arrived at the hospital considerably late. Fortunately, the hospital staff couldn't begin without us, since the star of the performance was in my care.

From this point on, everything went smoothly, and without incident. At precisely 9:39, we finally had some good news to share--a beautiful, healthy daughter. She had dark, almost black eyes, and since she had been brought into the world without any effort on her part, the perfect roundness of her tiny head was unscathed. She was even red-haired to blend in unobtrusively with her brother and sisters!

Gina's arrival momentarily took our minds off the invasion by Parkinson's. We were totally absorbed in the miracle of this new creation. Gina was a welcome reprieve from our troubles. Weighing in at 6 pounds, 14 ounces, she was perfect!

I was not permitted to escape reality for very long. When the nurse gently laid Gina in my arms, my entire body froze in sheer panic. How I wanted to caress and cuddle with her, to stroke her cheeks, count her fingers and toes--but I couldn't. All I could do was longingly stare at my new daughter, and tell her how much I loved her. Feeling completely inadequate at handling this overwhelming responsibility, I desperately wished someone would take Gina from me, fearful for her safety in my care.

The stress of surgery maximized my symptoms, and alarmed many uninformed staff throughout my hospital stay, necessitating an account of my problem. It was perhaps good practice, however, seeing their surprised and disturbed reactions. This was something I was going to witness quite often in the future.

One characteristic that is common among Parkinsonians is an unchanging, "masked" expression, which can be very misleading to people. It is particularly difficult to convey looks of enthusiasm, interest, or delight. I am often mistaken for being overly somber, bored, tired, worried, or depressed. To make matters worse, there is very little other body language on which to rely. When a message IS transmitted via body language, it is frequently an inaccurate message of fear or pain, falsely communicated by trembling, a frozen stature, or a cowering posture. I have learned to compensate for these discrepancies by either explaining this common mishap to people with whom I often converse, or by giving extra verbal clues to communicate my mood. These may or may not convince the listener.

This problem arose with a nursery attendant during my hospital stay. Because of the absence of research verifying the effects of antiparkinson drugs on breast feeding an infant, I chose to take the safe route and to feed Gina formula. To ease the disappointment, I determined to simulate the nursing experience as closely as possible. Since the bottle fed babies were routinely kept in the nursery throughout the night and fed by staff, I had to make my wishes known that Gina was to be brought to me for her nighttime feedings. The nursery attendant was a large, heavyset woman, with thick arms and man-sized hands. She had short, gray hair and a deep, intimidating voice of authority. The way that she confidently scooped Gina up and carried her to me on her hip--one-handed, like a football--told me that she had been caring for babies well before I even existed on this earth.

After timidly stating my request, the attendant frowned and shook her head disapprovingly. Seeing a shaky, languid mother with slouching shoulders, and no visible sign of life on her blank face, the attendant was adamant that I was making a grave mistake, and needed my rest. Only after I vehemently insisted, did she reluctantly comply with my demand.

Parkinson's disease has a strong tendency to make passive, compliant individuals out of its victims. It accomplishes this in two ways. First, by completely revamping the individual's self-image to include tremors, a shuffled gait, and garbled speech, the Parkinsonian is thoroughly stripped of his self-confidence. As a result, the afflicted adopt a timid, reticent nature, preferring to be inconspicuous, particularly in crowds and among strangers.

Secondly, compliancy is a conditioned response, acquired after a few encounters with the adverse effects of anger, excitement and fear on Parkinson's symptoms. Emotion at any intensity accentuates the unattractive traits of the disease. The Parkinsonian is quickly taught to build up a defense against this enemy called Emotion.

Even though I have become much more placid and reserved, there are those situations when my restraint gives way. Whenever possible, I choose the coward's method, and voice my anger via the phone or a letter. Unfortunately, this is not always a viable option. Issues involving what I perceive to be the best interests of my children, are most likely to invoke some strong feelings. I will often become uncharacteristically headstrong in my views. Arguing with the nursery attendant over my decision to feed Gina her nighttime bottles, myself, was such an instance!

The morning before my scheduled release from the hospital, a nurse roused me from a sound sleep, and wheeled me downstairs for the MRI brain scan. I had been dreading this test, ever since a friend had cautioned me about the possibility of feeling claustrophobic during the procedure. It was a great relief to discover that the MRI was not such an unpleasant experience after all.

It was obvious from the start that the technician was not accustomed to performing this test on patients who had just given birth by way of major surgery, when he instructed me to "hop" up onto the long narrow table and failed to offer any assistance! Barely able to rise up out of the wheelchair, I instantly called attention to his blunder. Lying on my back with my head inside a well-lit and mirrored magnetic tube, the technician kept me informed of each step throughout the procedure, using an intercom system. By preparing me for what was forthcoming, he eliminated a fear of the unknown, and allowed me to feel relatively calm and relaxed.

The MRI (Magnetic Resonance Imaging) is based on the premise that, normally, the protons in the body's atoms spin randomly around. The magnetic tube, however, forces the protons to align and spin in the same direction. A radio frequency signal is beamed into the tube, which moves the protons back out of alignment. When the signal stops, they realign and release energy. The scanner measures this energy and the time it takes for the protons to realign themselves. This information provides the radiologist with clues of possible tumors and diseases. The only annoyance during the entire procedure is a very loud tapping noise whenever the scanner is recording its findings. As expected, my test results came back normal.

The following morning, we hurriedly completed all the required paperwork for Gina's and my discharge from the hospital. Whereas I had often jokingly referred to my three previous maternity stays as "vacations," free from the responsibilities of cooking, cleaning and caring for the older children at home, this hospitalization had been a very draining experience-- hardly a vacation. I was particularly anxious this time for the comforts and privacy of home, and eager to reunite wih the rest of my family.

Andy, Becky and Stephanie also excitedly awaited our homecoming, impatient to meet their new sister. Even though they were not old enough to comprehend the magnitude of the problems we were facing, they sensed that they were needed. They were ready and willing to volunteer their services, and were immediately assigned tasks, fetching diapers and sleepers, or holding bottles. Our neighbors and church friends also came to our aid, providing many wonderful meals and cards of encouragement.

Even with all the support, I look back to much of Gina's first year in total awe, not having the vaguest idea how we managed to pull through this tumultuous period of our lives. In spite of the Sinemet, my movements were still extremely slow and clumsy, making it a struggle not only to feed and diaper Gina, but even to hold her. I fought to get a firm grip on her, and often panicked, as Gina would start slowly slipping through my fingers like a slick bar of wet soap. There were so many close calls. Everyone seemed very uneasy when I handled Gina, yet I could not bear to relinquish the job. Their distrust made me feel like the world's most incompetent mother. I dreaded the time spent alone with Gina.

I would often sadly recollect the days past, when I effortlessly adorned Becky or Stephanie in frilly dresses with big bows and teeny buttons, miniature tights, and tiny crocheted tie booties. Deprived of her femininity, Gina's attire, night or day, was limited to one-piece sleepers. It was challenge enough to tuck her clenched fist inside the sleeve's armhole, and sift through the opposite opening in search of that tiny fist. Once located, the tug of war began to straighten her bent arm, drawn stubbornly to her chest, in order to pull her hand completely down and through the sleeve. Fortunately, Gina was an exceptionally cheerful and even-tempered baby. I am certain God hand-picked her for us!

Contrary to my efforts to simplify my life by dressing Gina in sleepers, I stubbornly elected to use cloth diapers--pins, plastic pants, and all. Being conscientious about the environmental waste dilemma, as well as being staunchly opposed to the idea of throwing precious money out with every used paper diaper, I could not bear to use disposable diapers once our supply from gifts was depleted. Despite everyone's (including Paul's) inability to understand my obstinacy on the matter, I felt, and still feel, some positions are worth the extra effort. Even though I alone could not solve the landfill shortage problem, it certainly was not necessary for me to contribute to it. I washed, dried and pinned cloth diapers, putting two at a time on Gina, in order to cut down the number of changes necessary.

Six weeks after Gina's birth, I returned to Dr. Hastings for a reevaluation. Upon hearing my complaints, he prescribed an additional drug, Parlodel. Parlodel works quite differently than Sinemet. Sinemet contains levodopa, a substance which is used by the brain to produce the lacking chemical, dopamine. The dopamine then transmits messages between the neurons that govern movement. On the other hand, Parlodel is considered a "dopamine agonist". This class of drugs mocks the effects of dopamine by stimulating the dopamine receptors directly. Thus, they trick the brain into thinking it has received the dopamine, when in fact, it hasn't.

Within only two or three days after beginning the Parlodel, I was a new person. Or, perhaps, it is more accurate to say, I was my old self again. Whichever way you view it, it seemed like a miracle had occurred! The change was astonishing. My voice grew louder and clearer. My posture and gait returned to normal. All evidence of a tremor disappeared, and my coordination drastically improved. It was possible to laugh and smile once again. I was ecstatic and felt invincible! On this combination of Sinemet and Parlodel, I was experiencing what is known as the "levodopa honeymoon", the period of time, usually following the introduction of levodopa, when the patient receives the greatest response from the drug. The *honeymoon* typically lasts two or three years.

Life was perfect! I was symptom-free, except for those occasions when stress had the winning edge over the drugs. Thanksgiving that year was such a time. We celebrated the holiday at my brother-in-law's home in St. Louis. I was feeling especially thankful that day-- thankful for our new baby, for the miracle of medicine, and for the reprieve from the frustrating limitations of Parkinson's.

51--Parkinson's

Following the magnificent feast, we all gathered in the living room to visit. Moments later, I was distracted by a feud stirring between Stephanie and my three-year-old nephew, Joshua. Even though Stephanie was a mere twenty-three pounds at 2 1/2 years of age, she was small, but mighty. She had learned from living with an older sister and brother, to defend her rights. Maintaining a watchful eye, I chose to remain uninvolved in her dispute with Joshua, in hopes that my children will learn to iron out their own differences.

However, when Joshua reached over and grabbed Stephanie's arm, bearing his teeth and ready to make his attack, it was time to intervene! I lunged forward, screaming at the offender, as he chomped down on a mouthful of dress sleeve. Stephanie was spared, but the panic had triggered every Parkinson's symptom in me. Robbed of all the powers of the antiparkinson medicines, I was instantly shaky and rigid. It was almost an hour before I was able to regain my composure.

One afternoon, following the addition of Parlodel to my drug regimen, I became alarmed when my head jerked back, totally unpremeditated. Even though it appeared natural to the outer world, as if I were flinging my hair away from my face, I knew I was not in command! It was not long thereafter that a new word, "dyskinesia," was added to my rapidly enlarging vocabulary. Dyskinesias are involuntary extra movements--jerks and twitches, believed to be the result of over-stimulation within the nerve pathways regulated by dopamine. It is advisable to avoid this side effect for as long as possible, because the dyskinesias can eventually become as disabling as the disease itself.

Since I was already experiencing some dyskinesia, I questioned whether my current dosages of medication were too high, and desired a second opinion. Besides, being only thirty years old with a lifelong illness, I thought it would be wise to switch to a physician who specialized in Parkinson's disease in order to receive the optimal longterm care. I made a December appointment with a neurologist, Dr. Lee Tempel, affiliated with Washington University Medical School's Movement Disorders Clinic.

I was pleased to discover that Dr. Tempel was a young, ambitious doctor, dedicated to Parkinson's research. In the book, *Parkinson's: A Patient's View*, I recalled the author, Sidney Dorros, recommending that patients select a younger physician who will, hopefully, provide consistent medical care for the Parkinsonian for many years.[1]

Dr. Tempel also fit my criterion, in that he was conservative in prescribing, as well as increasing, medications. Most importantly, it was easy for me and Paul to talk with him. Dr. Tempel was willing to devote as much time as necessary to listen to our concerns, and to thoroughly answer all of our questions.

Choosing a physician whom I felt comfortable conversing with, and who seemed competent and well-versed on the subject of Parkinson's, was of the utmost importance to me. I was absolutely appalled at hearing one young man's story of his FORMER neurologist. Following his initial examination to determine the reason for his unexplained symptoms, the doctor had the audacity to call and leave a message on the patient's telephone answering machine, notifying him that his diagnosis was Parkinson's disease! Because the months preceding and following a C-section surgery and a new baby, are such an inopportune time to evaluate a patient's response to antiparkinson drugs, Dr. Tempel wanted to wean me off the Sinemet, and reserve this most potent drug for the future, if possible. He proposed I start over, this time on Parlodel alone. Cutting back on these medications can be a horrendous ordeal, as it often creates the "rebound effect". A patient may become much more symptomatic initially as dosages are reduced, before improving somewhat, and finally stabilizing at a certain level. The trick is remaining patient through the initial phase when symptoms are temporarily intensified. This is not an easy feat!

Despite Dr. Tempel's warning, it was very discouraging to lose all of my newly acquired skills. All of my old troubles recurred, the worst part being, that Gina was once again a struggle to hold. Needless to say, I became depressed. Although I had previously viewed depression as a personal weakness, I now knew it was out of my realm to control this indomitable feeling.

Depression frequently accompanies the symptoms of Parkinson's disease. As of yet, there are only theories as to why depression is so prevalent among Parkinsonians. Bouts of depression might be endogenous, resulting from chemical changes within the brain of the Parkinson's sufferer. Or, considering the high incidence of depression amongst all persons battling chronic illness, depression may be an emotional reaction to having a disability. Finally, it has been speculated that depression could be triggered by the medications used to treat Parkinson's disease. However, because depression existed in Parkinson's patients before the usage of today's antiparkinson drugs, this theory seems the least likely. It may be that a combination of factors cause depression.

Regardless of the cause, chronic depression is a concern that must be addressed. Contrary to the normal feelings of unhappiness pestering everyone from time to time, chronic depression persists, immobilizes, and rarely disappears untreated. Some of the criterion used in the diagnosis of clinical depression include:

* persistent feelings of sadness
* crying spells
* changes in appetite resulting
  in weight loss or weight gain
* problems with insomnia or hypersomnia
* feelings of worthlessness
* little or no energy
* difficulty concentrating and appearing less alert
* thoughts of death or suicide

It should be noted that some of these symptoms, such as changes in eating and sleeping habits, are characteristic of Parkinson's disease, and may not be indicative of depression. People suffering from chronic depression generally display a cluster of the above symptoms. Recalling the unyielding torment depression had created earlier in my life, I resolved to immediately confront it head on. Dr. Tempel suggested an antidepressant, amitriptyline. This particular tricyclic antidepressant has an anticholinergic effect, and could, therefore, possibly help my Parkinson's symptoms, in addition to elevating my mood. The loss of dopamine cells causes an imbalance in the brain with another neurotransmitter, acetylcholine, which is found in normal amounts in Parkinsonians. Instead of increasing the dopamine as Sinemet does, anticholinergics benefit the patient by hindering the work of the acetylcholine, and thus, helping to reinstate some of the balance. The amitriptyline did, in fact, make the period of rebounding more bearable for me.

Dr. Tempel experimented with various dosages of Parlodel over a five month period, before reinstating Sinemet, but at a smaller dosage than previously. The interminable demands of three small children and a baby called for more speed and coordination than I could muster from Parlodel alone.

With the return of Sinemet, the dyskinesias resumed, but this time, in the form of what I called "my happy feet". My feet were frequently overcome by an uncontrollable urge to tap dance, until I would stand up--at which time, the urge was somewhat subdued and my feet could regain their composure. My head no longer jerked, but started involuntarily nodding in perpetual agreement during the peak times of the medicines' cycles.

Even though we ended up back near square one and the experimentation had been very distressing at times, I feel it was imperative for Dr. Tempel to have tried different dosages and combinations, in order to find the minimal level of medication that would allow me to function reasonably well. Just as no two Parkinsonians are identical in their symptoms, so are they also different in the way that each responds to the antiparkinson medicines. A good doctor recognizes this factor, and approaches each patient with a "wait and see" attitude, as together, they work to find the best drug therapy.

By the end of my first year on antiparkinson medication, there was a well-established pattern to my days, which has basically continued to this day. In the morning I awaken, barely able to raise my voice above a whisper, and only able to walk with a distinct shuffle. Spontaneity is nonexistent, since I must methodically plot out my course of action before tackling even the simplest of tasks, such as opening a new box of Cheerios or untangling the twist tie on the bread bag-- motions which were completely taken for granted at one time in my life.

I am as dependent on my cherished pills to begin my day as other people are on their morning cup of caffeinated coffee. Waiting for the effects of my first dose of drugs of the day, I putter around, trying to motivate the children to move quickly, (unlike their mom!), at getting dressed and devouring their bowls of cereal. Approximately half an hour after ingesting those magic tablets, it is as if a light switch has suddenly been flipped on. I am off and running, accomplishing all that I can in an effort to take full advantage of this precious time, knowing that the allotted minutes are ticking away.

With the newly acquired agility, comes the emergence of dyskinesias. The dyskinesias spring up sporadically and without any advanced warning. In one respect, these jerks and twitches are almost a welcome relief, as they signal the temporary reprieve from the rigidity. However, as each month passes, these extra movements are becoming increasingly more intense, and longer lasting. Like the Parkinson's symptoms, the dyskinesias are intensified by stress and emotion.

I often allude to the dyskinesias as the acts of my pesty little ghost. At times the ghost is subdued and discreet, gently beckoning me to play with him by harmlessly tugging, prodding and tagging me. Being more of a nuisance than a hindrance, these movements are relatively easy to ignore.

At other times, though, the dyskinesias become an extremely irritating distraction, particularly when I am away from home and in a situation where I am expected to sit idly for extended periods of time, such as at a school or church meeting. On those occasions, the ghost, feeling rather frisky and intent on demanding my attention, resorts to roughly yanking, shoving, and thrusting me every which way--doing all in his power to antagonize me. Wrestling for control, I squirm, wiggle, twist and turn restlessly in my chair throughout the duration, much like a bored or an overly exuberant four-year-old. Unable to hold still for longer than a few seconds, I have tried sitting on my hands, wrapping my feet securely around the legs of my chair, and folding my arms, in an attempt to outwit the ghost. Despite my efforts, I have yet to meet with success. Fortunately, the ghost eventually grows weary and bored of the game, and leaves me in peace--at least until the next dose of medicine revives him!

My morning activities resemble any "normal" person's plans, with the exception of the dyskinesias. However, the spell is destined to break around the stroke of twelve. Unlike Cinderella, whose magic ended abruptly at twelve midnight, mine ceases around twelve noon. I also generally have more warning than Cinderella had, that my magic is ending. Usually, the Parkinson symptoms creep back in gradually. There are periodic surprises, though, when the magic from the pills is instantaneously replaced by the symptoms, leaving me feeling as if someone has just jerked the rug out from under my feet.

My attempts to time the next dose of drugs, so my forces will be armed and possibly able to deter the enemy, are sometimes successful. It requires precision timing so as not to take the pills too early, and thus, move the clock up on subsequent dosages. I do not want to deplete my resources and experience a power shortage before the close of day.

My second round of medicine works in much the same way as the first, losing its effectiveness near supper time. The third, and final, dose carries me through the major part of the evening. The next morning, the cycle repeats itself. Although the routine is fairly predictable, there is always that morning, afternoon, or evening when, for some inexplicable reason, the medicines totally fail to work, throwing a wrench into my plans. Over time, I have stumbled across a few clues as to how to get the most benefit from the pills, and avoid SOME of these wrenches. For instance, the drugs are most effective for me, and for many other Parkinsonians I have befriended along the way, if they are taken on an empty stomach. The levodopa in Sinemet is an amino acid. Amino acids are also the building blocks of the protein in food. The same carrier systems transport both the levodopa and certain amino acids in foods from the intestine to the bloodstream, and then to the brain. Therefore, when Sinemet is ingested at the same time as these amino acids, the levodopa must compete for the carrier in order to reach its final destination. Since levodopa can not work its magic until it enters into the brain, any delay means more "off" time for the Parkinsonian. There do exist some lucky people who can take levodopa with food, without having to relinquish any of the medicine's power. However, for many of us, it makes an almost inconceivable difference if Sinemet is taken prior to mealtimes, or on an empty stomach.

There are a few unfortunate souls whose systems can not tolerate the medicine without food, as nausea becomes a problem. One possible way to circumvent nausea may be to take supplemental tablets of carbidopa, a substance already contained in Sinemet to avert nausea, among other things.

Because of this rivalry between the levodopa in Sinemet and certain amino acids, many people have noted more favorable results when the antiparkinson drugs are not combined with a high protein diet. They have had to modify their menus and meal schedules, in order to get an adequate daily intake of protein, without interfering with their ability to function. The Recommended Dietary Allowance for protein is 0.8 grams/kilogram of body weight. After consulting with a physician or a dietician, many patients adhere to a special diet whereby foods rich in protein are avoided throughout the day, and reserved for the evening meal. By redistributing daily protein, many of Sinemet's daytime competitors are eliminated, and fluctuations in motor ability are not as drastic for certain people.

On the contrary, some research supports the theory that carbohydrates may actually provide a boost to levodopa's effectiveness. In fact, some physicians warn that meals high in carbohydrates MIGHT contribute to bouts of dyskinesia. I should note at this time that patients in the early stages of levodopa treatment are usually less sensitive to dietary factors. It is only after the passage of time that diet tends to play a more significant role in the management of Parkinson's disease.

Another way that I have discovered to maximize the effectiveness of the antiparkinson drugs is to time the dosages when I am not terribly anxious. Of course, these times are often totally unpredictable. Yet, there are many occasions when anxiety levels are expected to rise, such as the final fifteen minutes prior to making the mad rush out the door to go to church on Sunday mornings. Just about any time we are in the final preparations to leave home, and have to be somewhere at a designated time, is quite stressful. The more uptight I am feeling about needing the drugs to do their job, the more apt they are to be tardy.

Of course, the tips that work for me, may not apply to another Parkinsonian, and vice versa. A lot of knowledge is accumulated through a personal process of trial and error. Even with a wealth of information, Parkinson's has a way of surprising the patient with the unexpected and unexplainable change of plans, never allowing him to have full control over his life. However, by realizing the need to be flexible and learning how to roll with the punches, Parkinsonians can still retain the vantage point over their disease.

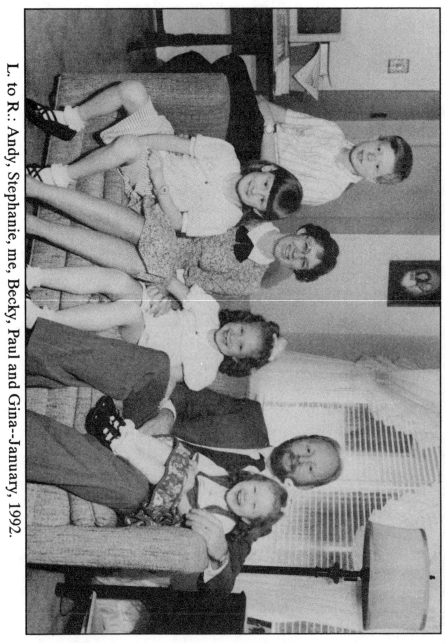

L. to R.: Andy, Stephanie, me, Becky, Paul and Gina–January, 1992.

Chapter 4
The Road to Acceptance

My acceptance of Parkinson's did not occur overnight. I first had to traverse the various stages of grieving that lead up to the final acceptance. After all, diagnosis of a chronic illness inevitably triggers grief-- grief over the loss of a normal life. My former dreams of the future had been devoid of tremors, neurologists, weekly trips to the pharmacist, dyskinesias, and wheelchairs. This drastic change in plans necessitated a mourning period. It takes time to sort out emotions, and to assess both blessings and obstacles, in preparation for forging ahead with life.

Renown psychiatrist, Elisabeth Kubler-Ross, in her landmark book, *On Death and Dying*, outlines five stages of the grieving process: denial, anger, bargaining, depression, and acceptance.[2] Dr. Kubler-Ross proposes that the different stages do not always evolve separately and in the order specified above. Although her views were formulated with the terminally ill person in mind, I can easily see applicability to others who are grieving, for whatever reason.

As I was bemoaning deprivation of a healthy future, I partook in each of the five stages along the road to acceptance. I did not always adhere to the classical sequence, and sometimes, reverted back to a stage I had already passed through. In fact, to this day, I still find myself ricocheting back and forth among some of the stages during moments of fear or frustration.

The first stage, denial, was likewise my initial phase of the process. Possessing an indestructible determination to deny the onset of a serious problem, I clung desperately to every means of escaping the truth. I worked diligently to convince myself that the symptoms were sensory nerve damage, anxiety, stress-- anything but reality. No one could persuade me otherwise.

Although I blindly groped through the denial stage prior to the actual diagnosis, many Parkinsonians I've met experienced their denial period afterward, ardently refusing to accept their doctor's definitive conclusion. Yet, still other people affirm the diagnosis but deny the serious ramifications that the disease entails. Parkinson's becomes an inescapable part of one's daily life. It is overly simplistic to declare that life will go on as before. I do not mean to imply that Parkinsonians should not have a positive, undefeated attitude with the determination to continue striving and succeeding. They must, however, expect life to change, and adapt accordingly.

I still periodically drift in and out of the anger stage of the grieving process. I have never lingered in a state of anger for any great length of time, perhaps, because I am not, by nature, a hot tempered person. Yet, I have felt anger momentarily, particularly toward individuals who fail to recognize their countless blessings in life. For whatever reason, they can not rejoice in living and relish each day. It is amazing how trivial the complaints of my friends now seem, complaints that I too shared at one time. It is a shame everyone can not step in the shoes of a Parkinsonian for one day, and know firsthand how it feels to shake uncontrollably in the check-out line at the grocery store, with a dozen pairs of eyes gazing at you in bewilderment. Or realize how it feels to battle 45 minutes just to make one pony tail in the hair of your impatient and wiggly four year old daughter. Or experience how it feels to wake up in the morning and only be able to whisper a faint, garbled "good morning" to your spouse. Or understand how helpless it feels to hear your baby screaming hysterically, and not be able to work your unresponsive fingers underneath her to secure a firm grip, so you can cuddle her in your arms to comfort her. It would change their whole perspective on life! Imagining is not equivalent to experiencing.

Ironically, these are many of the same uninformed people whose choice words of solace upon learning of my impaling diagnosis were, "Well, it could be worse." I always felt like shouting in retort, "Well, it could be better!" Unfortunately, MOST people do not know the appropriate and most soothing response to distressing news. Contrary to popular belief, a grieving person is not appeased by such statements as, "It is all for a reason", "God has a plan for you", "We should praise God for everything", or "God never gives us more than we can handle." (If I'd have known, I would have appeared less capable!) Rather, a lamenting person desires only a silent hug, or to hear simply, "I'm sorry." People should not feel compelled to provide an explanation, or to downplay the person's sorrow, but instead, allow them time to hurt. Most likely, I also had some repressed anger toward God. Why had God allowed this to happen to me, or had He? Why did Parkinson's disease have to be included in His grand master plan for my life, or was it? Everyone formulates their own image of God, and His role in our lives, based on their personal experiences. Some people's perceptions of God never change, for they never have experiences that challenge their personification of Him. However, mine had been rivaled by Parkinson's, and had not withstood the test. It was necessary to reconsider my pre-Parkinson's image of God, and His involvement in our earthly lives.

After diligently searching for answers to my questions through reading and conferring with others, my relationship with God has grown. I understand Him differently now. I strongly affirm that God did not "give" me or plan for me, or anyone else, to develop Parkinson's, or to encounter any other crisis in life. God is too loving a parent to wish suffering on His children, but He also does not shelter us from life, though He may want to. God did not make us to be manipulated puppets. Rather, He created free creatures, free to make our own choices in life--EVEN the choice to act for or against God, Himself. When He created us, He equipped us with all that we would need for living in this world. He left it up to us to seek out and use these copious resources. However, that does not mean that we no longer need God, or that He can't affect our futures. God remains ever present for us as our spiritual advisor, a resource that can drastically affect how we handle the ups and downs of life on this earth.

So why do I have Parkinson's? I can only speculate on the answer to that question. Perhaps we, as a society, made poor choices along the way, and polluted the environment with a toxin that triggers Parkinson's in certain people. Whatever the cause, I believe that when I was crying in sorrow from the stabbing news of my diagnosis, God was right there, crying alongside me just as any caring parent would be. God stood ready to render His spiritual guidance to lead me onward, if I asked Him for it. Because I did turn to Him, God has furnished me with tremendous strength and has shown me how to creatively use my suffering to live a meaningful life.

Kubler-Ross cites bargaining as the third step in grieving. Bargaining involves negotiating an agreement with someone, possibly God. I passed through this stage simultaneously with my phase of denial and tremendous fear, before my actual diagnosis. Probably, I was engaging in subliminal bargaining with God when I began teaching Sunday school, ringing bells, and reading the Bible daily. I subconsciously deemed that if I faithfully served God, He would return the favor and rid me of my problems.

Depression often follows bargaining. Depression erroneously creates the illusion that you are the only one suffering; that life has unjustly sentenced you, and you alone, with an affliction. This feeling fosters self-pity. In actuality, though, we unknowingly come in daily contact with people who are hurting just as deeply. No one is immune to misfortune.

I was enrolled in a mini-course at church, which involved sharing our tribulations with the group. As we each revealed our current personal struggles, it was obvious that I was facing the most serious hardship. Everyone else's problems seemed so minute in comparison.

Two weeks after the course ended, one woman from the class was struck with the piercing news that she had massive breast cancer. This was the same person who, two weeks before, had cited her unsold house as her greatest trial. Suddenly my cross seemed lighter.

It is only natural that a newly diagnosed Parkinsonian should experience depression. Many of their dreams and goals in life are dashed, and must be altered or forgotten. My heart had been set on being an actively involved mother, participating in scouts, P.T.A., church activities, etc. Eventually I had hoped to resume my teaching career. I had envisioned my retirement years with Paul, enjoying travel, and the freedom to do as we pleased. Even though I have been forced to let go of many of my aspirations, I have discovered over time, new challenges to keep my life purposeful.

My most effective strategy for working through this phase of depression, is talking with others. Upon receiving my diagnosis, I had a tremendous craving to pour out my feelings and thoughts on anyone and everyone. I probably did not need to hear what they had to say, as much as I needed to talk--to unload and share some of the burden I was holding within. Unfortunately many people avoided or diverted the topic, seeing how painful it was for me, and unaware that I needed, and wanted, to disperse some of this pain. On one occasion, I sent a thank-you to a circle of church friends, who had furnished my family with a wonderful dinner soon after Gina's birth. In the note, I stressed that the group could feel free to speak with me about Parkinson's, even if it prompted tears, explaining that sometimes I needed to cry. Later, several friends shared with me how meaningful my letter had been for them.

The final destination--acceptance. Acceptance does not mean I have passively resigned myself to the fact that I have Parkinson's disease, and must bravely endure the consequences. Instead, acceptance implies that I have become well-informed on the subject of Parkinson's disease, so that my symptoms can be best managed. There are so many ways to minimize the Parkinson's, and maximize the drugs' effectiveness. Acceptance does not eliminate the need to hope for a cure, either. Rather, it intensifies the need, and stirs me into action toward finding that cure.

One of the easiest, and most effective ways to become knowledgeable about Parkinson's, is by joining a support group. Parkinsonians have the edge on doctors, even neurologists, when it comes to understanding certain (but not all!) aspects of the disease. They also have the most comprehensive list of coping techniques. Doctors are limited to what they can observe, read, or speculate. The Parkinsonian acquires his knowledge from living with the disease day and night.

Parkinson's disease affects a vast, and growing number of people. It is estimated that there are 1.5 million sufferers in the United States alone. There are more Parkinson's victims than there are people diagnosed with multiple sclerosis, muscular dystrophy, and A.L.S. (amyotrophic lateral sclerosis) combined. [3] Yet, there are still many misconceptions concerning Parkinson's, even within the medical community. It is ideal to collect information through reading up-to-date literature, finding a competent and current physician, and collaborating with a few of those 1.5 million experts. Parkinsonians and their spouses, or other significant partners, who study the disease 24 hours a day, and 365 days a year, are a key resource.

Support groups house a wealth of valuable information. Conversation is never at a loss at these meetings. Support groups are also safe and nonjudgemental places where the Parkinsonian and his/her partner can confide a host of esoteric experiences, concerns, fears and frustrations. The common bond linking the members, instantly fosters friendships.

In January of 1989, four months after learning that I had Parkinson's disease, Paul and I attended a local support group for Parkinsonians and their partners. We both desperately needed to converse with others who were facing the same challenges.

Although the next youngest person in the room was a woman twice our age, it was still beneficial to hear the group discussing many of the same issues with which we were dealing. Since we had additional problems that needed to be addressed, and because the 10:00a.m. meeting time conflicted with Paul's job, we decided to form our own support group geared toward Parkinsonians under 55 years of age.

Our first task was to find someone willing to facilitate the group. That was easy. One of my closest friends, Renee Kirschbaum, had an undergraduate degree in social work, and a master's degree in counseling. As hoped, she readily agreed to fill the position.

Because we had planned to hold the monthly meetings in our own home, the next task on the agenda was to locate some interested participants. We contacted Susan Levin, the Parkinson's Disease Information and Referral Center coordinator in St. Louis. She enthusiastically agreed to publish a notice, announcing the formation of our new group, in the *St. Louis Parkinson Newsletter*. Paul and I also publicized the group in a community journal, and on fliers. The fliers were displayed on various grocery store and library bulletin boards.

Although response was initially slow, our support group got off the ground with its first meeting on April 3, 1989, with a total of six people. For three hours we chattered incessantly, sharing stories of our initial diagnoses, names of our physicians, types and amounts of medicines being taken, etc. It was a very upbeat discussion. Everyone left that evening, feeling encouraged and comforted by the realization that they were no longer alone in their battle. Despite the small turnout, the meeting was a success!

As word of our group spread and the size increased, Paul and I were continually stunned by the unpredictable nature of Parkinson's disease. No two people are affected in the same way. Some symptoms may NEVER surface in certain individuals, and the rate of progression is just as indiscriminate. This revelation caused Paul to begin referring to Parkinson's as "a very political disease," for there are never any straight answers on the subject.

Within the first year of its existence, the support group outgrew our home. With approximately 25 members, it continues to reach even more people today. Drawing from the expertise of the members, and periodically an outside speaker, we have gleaned invaluable information and ideas on managing Parkinson's, which are shared throughout this book.

Most importantly, we have established some special friendships within the group--friends who can relate to the aggravation of trying to get on a knife that last evasive dab of peanut butter, stuck to the center of the bottom of the jar. Or friends who know firsthand the frustration of losing your own hand in the deep chasm of your pocket while weaving in and out of the mountainous folds of fabric in search of an elusive coin. Or friends who can identify with the battle of breaking through all the extra packaging--the cellophane wrapper, the glued box, the child-proof lid (or, more accurately, the Parkinsonian-proof lid!), the safety seal, and the enormous wad of cotton--just to get to the imprisoned Tylenol! Or those who can empathize with the challenge of trying to mentally command those rebellious fingers to scrub hard and fast enough to work up a lather of shampoo on their heads. Or friends who can truly understand the predicament of being trapped in the sheets of their own bed. It is similar to the plight of a fly, which, after being ensnared in the web of a spider, is bound motionless.

A common rebuttal against the necessity of participating in a support group, is the argument that exposure to more progressed patients can be too depressing and frightening. I must truthfully confess that it can be disturbing, particularly to a recently diagnosed Parkinsonian or his spouse, to be confronted with wheelchair-bound persons or extremely symptomatic or dyskinetic individuals. But once you venture forth and risk becoming acquainted with them, you begin to see beyond the wheelchair, the wildly thrashing and flailing arms, the whisper of unintelligible speech, or the drunken gait. Instead, you see the real person, with a witty sense of humor, a contagious courage, or an inspiring view on life. Parkinsonians, even the most advanced patients, have much to offer others. Avoiding these people only stagnates an individual in the denial stage, and robs them of an opportunity to gain some treasured friendships.

Because I attest that acceptance involves sufficiently educating yourself on the disease, as well as becoming active in the search for a cure, it follows that a healthy level of acceptance also includes a willingness to confide the diagnosis with others. By openly admitting that I have Parkinson's to friends, and even strangers I encounter, it affords me the opportunity to educate more individuals on the disability, and thus, enlist more supporters to my worthy cause--securing a cure. When others are aware of my problem, it reduces stress, an enemy of the Parkinsonian. I once spoke on the telephone with a young man who had coped, virtually alone, for ten years with Parkinson's. He was obstinately opposed to unveiling his disability to anyone. He painfully recollected the abashment and chagrin he had once felt while serving on a jury. The selected jurors had been assigned to a tragic case involving a child, who had been accidentally killed by a garbage truck. As the jurors were passing the gruesome pictures of the accident, the young man had been overcome by an uncontrollable tremor throughout his body. Unwilling to explain that his shaking was due to Parkinson's disease, and had been instigated by the stress of the case, he was promptly dismissed from his duties. Shot down by humiliation and embarrassment, he exited the room in discomposure. How much easier to have been frank about his illness!

Trying to hide the Parkinson's from those around us, consumes a great deal of energy, as well as increases stress levels. No matter how well concealed the symptoms appear to the Parkinsonian, other people may still question (not necessarily aloud) certain peculiar mannerisms, peering out from under the guise.

One bright sunny morning in the summer of 1989, soon after Dr. Tempel had decided to start me again on the Sinemet, I woke up feeling especially chipper. Finally noticing the effects of the Sinemet on my symptoms, I was ready to tackle anything. Feeling like "Wonder Woman," I loaded all four children in the van, buckled them in their seats, and headed for the grocery store. Grocery shopping with three children and a baby--a piece of cake! As I strolled up and down the aisles, I marveled at how inconspicuous I surely appeared, looking just like every other mom--normal! With my cart crammed to the max, I proceeded toward the check-out. I was on the homestretch now!

Since it was a store policy to offer customer assistance to the car, the bagger politely offered to accompany me outside, once the final bag had been wedged in my cart. Rationalizing that there were three children on foot to keep tabs of in the parking lot, I gratefully accepted her help. We were nearing the van when the bagger glanced over and timidly asked, "Are you OK? You look sick." It was as though I were a soaring kite, and suddenly the wind had ceased blowing. As I did a nosedive for the ground, I smiled weakly and replied, "Yes, I'm fine. I just have Parkinson's disease." It suddenly occurred to me that I no longer knew what it felt like to be "normal".

Except in that rare instance when it may jeopardize one's job, I recommend being up front with people. Virtually everyone I have encountered has been receptive and understanding. John Holland, a truly inspiring man, had struggled for ten years with Parkinson's, at the time we met. He shared with me a business-sized card that he carries with him for distribution to clerks, cashiers, etc. The card reads:

> I have Parkinson's Disease
> It is *not* contagious, a mental
> condition, hereditary, or
> fatal. It is a movement
> disorder.
>
> Because of this, I may need
> extra time to communicate
> and/or transact business
> with you.
>
> Thank you for your
> patience.

Another method of silently communicating a disability is by wearing a medical ID bracelet. Not only does it catch the public's eye, but it is also a worthwhile investment in the event of an emergency. It instructs people that I have Parkinson's, and furnishes the name of my doctor. I would not want to be hospitalized for an emergency without passing along this pertinent information. No telling what complication they might mistakenly treat me for! I also would not want to go any length of time without receiving my cherished antiparkinson drugs.

Acceptance of Parkinson's disease takes time, but everyone reaches this optimal stage in the grieving process, if that is their aim. Sure, some days I feel very depressed or angry. But most of the time I accept my illness, remembering what a dear friend, Curt Ballard, once said to me. "You know, a cure may be as close as tomorrow."

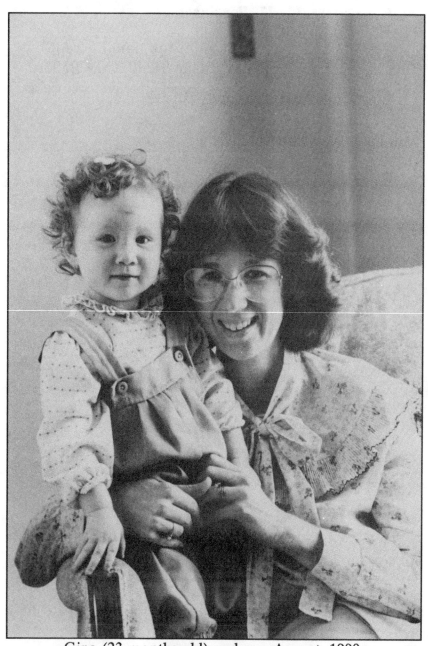

Gina (23 months old) and me--August, 1990.

Chapter 5
A Family Affair

I often worried about how my children would fare, growing up with a mother who has Parkinson's disease. Children learn so much through imitation of those around them, and I was their key model, with my own unique style of doing certain skills. It especially troubled me that Gina would never know me without the Parkinson's. What influence would my poor speech patterns have on Gina as she learned to talk? Would she acquire fine motor coordination without my example? How would it affect all four of my children to be nurtured by a seemingly solemn, unhappy mother, who rarely laughed or smiled?

Whereas children with disabled parents need to have a surplus of patience, I think they instinctively acquire the necessary amounts. Instead, I will venture to guess that the most difficult aspect of being reared by a parent who has Parkinson's is the lack of facial expression and body language. Interpreting emotions, without any visual clues, requires a great deal of insight into people and/or an understanding of the disability. It is tricky enough for adults to compensate, but children, especially, are not adept at reading between the lines.

Becky is my extra sensitive child, frequently seeking approval from those around her. More than once, I can recall her peering up with those big, blue, serious eyes, her face framed by long, red banana curls, and asking me, in a most concerned voice, "Mommy, why are you so sad?" Each time, it nearly broke my heart to realize I was inadvertently conveying this message to her. These episodes have impressed on me the importance of providing my children with frequent reminders that my failure to smile or laugh is due to the Parkinson's, and not because I am sad. Now, understanding that a stern face does not necessarily reflect my mood, Becky serves as my constant reminder, regularly ordering me to "Smile, Mom!"

I have also learned to verbalize my inner feelings, rather than to expect my children to rely solely on deceptive or lacking visual clues. Even an affirmative nod to a child's query can be misleading. At times my head bobs incessantly much like those dogs in car windows whose heads are attached by a spring. My head may say "yes", but my answer may be "no". Having grown accustomed to the incongruities, my children often press for verbal confirmation to determine if approval was truly granted, before forging ahead with an idea.

On the other side of the fence, the most difficult aspect, for me, of being a parent with Parkinson's, has been redefining the characteristics of a "good" parent. Intellectually, I know it is entirely possible to do an adequate, and even a superb job of parenting, with this disability. Still, it has been a tremendous struggle for me to emotionally accept this idea. My image of a "good" mother formerly consisted of active involvement in all those activities which require time, energy, coordination, and a tolerance for stress. I envisioned myself whipping up cookies for P.T.A. meetings, sewing elaborate Halloween costumes for my children, and volunteering to help with church Christmas pageants. Since these activities could not always be arranged in accordance with my "on" and "off" times, I had to reconsider my expectations of a "good" parent. Reevaluating my job description has not been easy to do, especially when surrounded by friends who are scout leaders, classroom aides, and volunteer drivers for school field trips. Plus, I am bombarded daily by the media with explicit instructions on how to be the perfect parent. Magazines feature articles titled "Twelve Tips to Develop A Positive Self-Esteem in Your Child". Radio and television talk shows interview prominent psychologists who have written entire books on how to create a stimulating environment for your infant, toilet train your toddler, insure school success for your five-year-old, and communicate with your teenager. My children have even brought home fliers from school publicizing an eight week course on "Successful Parenting". Although there may be a lot of helpful information to be gained from these resources, they fail to address the parent whose dyskinesias interfere with his ability to throw a ball to his youngster, the parent whose waning, garbled speech makes it difficult to hold the attention of a child through the reading of a classic storybook, and the parent whose trembling hands impede his ability to assist with a delicate school project. The discouragement of not being able to live up to all these expectations has led me to rely primarily on my instincts. I have had to focus exclusively on the other means of communicating love to my children--ways which are still within my capabilities, such as being an attentive listener when my children have things to share, or giving them a healthy self-esteem by allowing them the pride from doing things for themselves.

As a parent with Parkinson's, I also struggle with the tendency of misdirecting anger at my children--anger which was actually intended for my symptoms. My children often unknowingly stumble into the line of fire, and become innocent victims. Such a time might be when Stephanie has inquisitively asked "Why?" for the tenth consecutive time at a moment when my mouth feels as though it is wired shut, and talking is a wearisome job. Or when I am just seconds away from the victory of sliding that tiny button through the equally tiny buttonhole, and Becky innocently fidgets, causing me to lose my grip and have to start over from scratch. Or when I have painstakingly sorted and folded a load of laundry only to discover later that Gina has dismantled in fifteen seconds that which took me fifteen minutes to complete!

All parents wrongly snap at their children from time to time when stress prevails over their patience. I am just more susceptible since stress presides in almost every task I undertake, from signing my name on a check to refolding an empty grocery bag. My patience barely has a fighting chance against the overpowering forces of stress.

However, there is also the reverse problem in regards to anger. Anger has a reputation for riling up either Parkinson's symptoms or dyskinesias. Having experienced the hazards of allowing Anger to take the platform and speak its peace, I sometimes choose the gutless alternative and muzzle the troublemaker. Consequently, my children often escape a deserved verbal reprimand, and discipline is inconsistent. When I do accept the challenge to deliver a necessary scolding to one of my cherubs, it is difficult to be effective if Anger forms a comraderie with Parkinson's. It is an arduous task to convey anger to a child with a soft, unconvincing voice, a calm, unperturbed face, a gentle, unintimidating grip of his arm, and a waning supply of energy. Yet, despite my struggles with playing the role of firm disciplinarian, I have been blessed with four generally well-behaved, respectful children--adept at recognizing my covert anger.

All things considered, children are more resilient and discerning than we often expect. Most of my initial worries over parenting with Parkinson's have since been dismissed. Needless to say, Gina did learn to speak, and with very clear, intelligible articulation, well ahead of schedule. And her quick mastery of puzzles demonstrated her acquisition of fine motor coordination. And finally, not one of my four children have adopted a somber disposition. All of these things--despite my influence!

Children continually surprise adults with their capacity to grasp problems affecting their family, and to deal with them remarkably well. Gina recently demonstrated her keen perceptiveness, as well as her atypical vocabulary for a 2 1/2-year-old. Paul and I were the co-chairpersons for the 1991 Parkinson's Disease Walk-A-Thon sponsored by the St. Louis Chapter of the American Parkinson Disease Association. During one of the weekly organizational meetings at our home, I excused myself to herd the children off to bed. Feeling impatient with the girls' never ending ploys to procrastinate bedtime, I hurriedly planted one last kiss on each forehead and sternly reminded them that I needed to return to my meeting. Gina sprang up in her bed and inquisitively murmured through her pacifier, "Meeting?...Parkazeez?" Even though Paul and I had never spoken directly with her concerning Parkinson's disease, Gina had somehow acquired a sense as to where it fit in the scheme of things.

If information about Parkinson's is shared with children in a positive and sensitive way, they will develop a favorable and hopeful sentiment about the disability. Sheltering children from this reality is not in their best interest. Parkinson's is undeniably a "family disease", affecting every member of the household. Thus, children need to be included in an open discussion to allay fears, resolve puzzlement, and instruct them on ways they can be most helpful. It is imperative to realize that children attain acceptance through mimicking their parents' undefeated attitude.

Becky has clearly accepted my disability as a simple fact of life--almost a privilege! At the last meeting before the Walk-A-Thon, Becky sat perched on my lap, munching her popcorn and absorbing all the final preparations being made. Forgetting her place as a silent observer, she leaned over the table to establish eye contact with an unsuspecting committee member. Curiosity having gotten the best of her, Becky inquired of him, "Do you have Parkinson's disease?" Upon receiving a disappointing "No", Becky sighed, "Well, SOMEONE should!"

Children may or may not need to grieve after learning that their parent has Parkinson's. Their reaction will depend on their age, their nature, how the news is presented to them, and how those around them are coping. Just as adults are entitled to their grief, children should not be deprived of their feelings, including anger and depression. Parents need not intervene unless a child is mired in a particular stage, unable to move on unassisted.

Andy was seven years old when I received my diagnosis. It was not long afterward that I resolved to inform Andy of our unfortunate news. Because of his youthfulness, the discussion had to be kept simple and encouraging. I wanted to be particularly careful not to plant any detrimental fears.

Our chat began with a brief definition of the illness, Parkinson's disease, in terms which Andy could comprehend. I cited unusual mannerisms that he had possibly observed in me, and explained that these were the result of the Parkinson's. This was the reason why my hands shook, why I often spoke too softly or unclearly, and why it took me so long to complete tasks, such as making his lunch, or getting a knot out of his shoe string. I was also mindful to clarify the reason I needed to take so much medication.

To ensure that he did not harbor any unspoken fears or concerns, I made a point to explicitly assure Andy that Parkinson's disease was not fatal, and that I did not contract it because of anything he, or anyone else, had done. I explained that no one knew the cause of the disease. Since there currently is no cure for Parkinson's, I recruited Andy's support in helping us do our part to find one.

Several months later, it became apparent that one other pertinent piece of information had been overlooked during our talk. One brisk autumn afternoon, Andy shuffled wearily through the door from outside, where he had been playing with neighborhood friends. His cheeks were flushed and hot, and he complained that his head ached. It didn't take a quick thinker to deduce that he had a virus of some kind. As I grabbed the afghan from the couch to cover him, and began vigorously shaking down the thermometer, Andy sighed, and nonchalantly suggested, "Maybe I am getting Parkinson's disease, Mom. I have been around you a lot lately." It instantly struck me that I had failed to mention during our prior discussion, that Parkinson's is not contagious. Fortunately, the subject had been presented in such a calm and positive way, that it did not seem as if Andy had been worrying needlessly over the possibility of catching Parkinson's. Even when the thought crossed his mind, Andy's attitude appeared to be one of resigned acceptance.

Although Paul and I were openly and freely discussing Parkinson's in the presence of all of our children, we neglected to sit down and conference individually with the girls early on, as I had done with Andy. We mistakenly assumed they were too young to understand at the naive ages of 3 and 4 years, and so we had postponed their discussions. We probably underestimated them, though, and I would recommend that even children this young be given some explanation. Many preschool-aged children are old enough to absorb the gist of the situation. They are also old enough, however, to formulate misconceptions based on bits of conversation they have overheard. By initiating a brief discussion of Parkinson's with them, many misunderstandings can be prevented, as youngsters will feel free to voice their concerns, and pose their questions.

Once we opened the door for discussion, it has been intriguing to listen to our children's questions, and observe their minds at work as they sort through our answers, trying to make sense of this puzzling thing called "Parkinson's". They have addressed such issues as why I don't smile, why I am so "wiggly", why my hands "look old", why I "look mad", and if I will die from Parkinson's. The most popular question, though, has been "How did you get Parkinson's?" Dissatisfied with my plea of ignorance, they reinterrogate me every month or so, searching for a better response. I suspect the underlying reason for my children's unwaning interest in the cause of Parkinson's is that they host a fear of contracting the disease, themselves. "How did you get Parkinson's?" is my children's way of asking "Will I get Parkinson's, too?"

After the facts were shared with Becky and Stephanie, they put forth more effort at stifling their demands, and allowed me extra leeway. It was helpful that they could attach a reason to my slowness. On those occasions when the girls forget and impatiently make five urgent requests of me at once, I need only to gently remind them, "You must be patient. I have Parkinson's disease, and can not move that quickly." This usually curtails their nagging.

In addition to educating my children at their appropriate levels of understanding, developing a sense of humor about the situation has also been extremely beneficial. This is true for Paul and me, as well. I will always remember when Gina was about ten months old. She was entering that adorable stage when babies learn to wave by mimicking their caretakers. (At least, it is adorable to the child's parents.) With me as her primary teacher, Gina mastered what we later termed her "Parkinsonian wave". Rather than laxly waving her hand at the wrist, Gina had learned to wave by stiffly and mechanically moving her entire arm up and down! She looked like a marionette with an invisible string attached to her hand, which was yanked up and down by the puppeteer upon receiving the cue to wave.

Bill Heitman, a very bright and witty man in our support group, has encouraged his children, by his example, to seek out the humor in his predicament. One sizzling Fourth of July, Bill's family joined our crew for a picnic, and to view a spectacular air show.

89--Parkinson's

Bill was having a frustrating day controlling his symptoms. The extreme heat was probably not helping matters. Bill spent the entire afternoon either completely rigid like a motionless scarecrow, or very dyskinetic, with his arms, legs and head thrashing in perpetual motion. The sponsors of the show opened several fire hydrants so the spectators could cool off from the steamy 105 degree temperature. Two of Bill's children, aged ten and twelve, asked permission of their father to leave our spot and take refuge in the water for a while. Bill was wrestling a bout of dyskinesias at the time. He was writhing and rolling sporadically on a blanket spread out on the ground. He resembled a nervous fish taken from the security of its home in the water.

Gaining their dad's approval, the two children started to trot merrily off toward the crowd of people, who were already drenching themselves. Bill piped out one last word of advice, "Don't talk to any weirdos along the way--unless, of course, it's your father!"

Bill was equally good-natured that day when Gina, who was then one and a half years old, stared--mystified, at his dyskinetic movements. His body was gyrating and swaying, his head nodding rhythmically to the silent beat, and his fingers moving, as if they were playing an invisible piano. Suddenly Gina grinned with apparent understanding, and then began dancing along with Bill!

My children have become unusually self-sufficient, caring, and responsible individuals because of our unique household. Paul's and my favorite story, illustrating their commendable independence, stars our middle daughter, Stephanie. Stephanie sensed, at the tender age of three, that she was needed, and a vital contributor to our family.

One evening, we were chattering away about the day's events, as we gobbled down our dinner. Gina was contently confined to her wind-up baby swing in the corner of the living room. I was oblivious to her needs, and to those of our dog, Cinnamon, who was sitting patiently at the back door, whining softly, in hopes of someone letting her outside. I was totally engrossed in eating and talking until Stephanie instinctively popped up out of her chair and marched straight for the back door. Without hesitation, she unlocked the door, opened it, and reached outside for the dog's chain. Then, after hooking Cinnamon up, she closed and securely locked the door before circling back to the kitchen. On her way, she noticed Gina sitting motion-less in her swing. Stephanie detoured across the room, thoughtfully cranked up the swing, gave Gina a gentle push, and proceeded back to her place at the table. Without saying a word or expecting any gratitude, she continued eating her dinner. Paul and I stared at one another in disbelief. We had one very capable three-year-old!

Even Gina, when she was only a couple of months old, was already striving to become self-sufficient. During her infancy, I was still in the experimental stage with medications and dosages. Much of this time, my level of functioning was less than tolerable. Whenever

Gina was lying flat on her back on the floor or in her crib, fussing for some attention, it was a real struggle for me to secure a firm grip before lifting her. It often felt as if my hands were not attached to my body. I could not seem to relay messages from my brain to my fingers, instructing them to cooperate, and squeeze under Gina's back, firmly grasp her sides, and lift up. Instead, I had to carefully calculate my every move. Eventually, just like Pavlov's dog, Gina became conditioned. As soon as I would reach to pick her up, her conditioned response was to raise her head up off the floor or crib! She knew what came next. We joked that she was silently cheering me on, "You can do it, Mom! Go for it! I'll help you!"

Our children are also acquiring admirable confidence and determination that, where there is a will, there is a way. Experience has taught them that if you want something done quickly, don't ask Mom, particularly if fine motor coordination is involved. Becky quickly learned Mom was not the person to put the skimpy dress on her Barbie doll. Nor was Mom the one to fasten the four tiny buttons down the back of her dress. And Mom was certainly not the one to braid her long curly hair! It was far better to recruit someone else's help. Anyone else would do--a sister or brother, her Dad, or even a guest, visiting our home. And, if there were no other available choices, Becky would attempt, and frequently succeed at teaching herself to do the job. All my children mastered their self-help skills at far younger ages than the norm because of my disability. The problem arises when they began assuming that no task is beyond their capabilities, such as when two-year-old Gina attempted to pour a gallon jug of milk to get herself a drink! My family has also acquired phenomenal listening skills. Their remarkably keen ears can detect and decipher my faint, wispy mutters from across a noisy room when no one else present even realizes I have spoken. My children must frequently serve as translators for me to their friends.

I must confess that my children's table manners have probably suffered because of my Parkinson's. When I am functioning at my worst, I have a tendency to bring my mouth down to the food, rather than the food up to my mouth. I also slurp the milk directly from the cereal bowl, instead of painstakingly dishing it out, one spoonful at a time. I often eat with a spoon even when proper etiquette calls for the use of a fork. It is far less time consuming to scoop up with a spoon than to try to corner and stab those slick, evasive peas with a fork, or to balance slippery spaghetti noodles on the high wires of the fork from plate to mouth. Finally, when there is no company for dinner, I use my fingers to grab a handful of lettuce salad, and plop it on each plate, rather than wrestle with those awkward and uncooperative salad tongs. Yet, my children will likely survive, as long as Emily Post does not accompany us for dinner!

Even though our children are more independent, more caring toward others, and more responsible than the average child, we have learned that they have a limit to how much independence and responsibility they can reasonably handle. It is very easy to rely excessively on them, and to expect too much from them. Children still need to be children, with carefree time to run and play.

The year prior to and the year following my diagnosis, I was frantically trying to manage the household. Andy was so easy going and competent, that I began depending on his help. He readily assumed the role of caregiver, as he was called upon to entertain Gina for brief intervals, to fetch unreachable toys or clothes for Becky or Stephanie, to clean up after his sisters, and to run errands for me. Paul followed suit with additional requests. Nothing we asked of him was beyond his capabilities, but all of the chores compiled were overwhelming for him.

Andy's mounting frustration was not visible at home. He always agreeably complied with our wishes. However, during both his kindergarten and first grade years, the teachers' reports were identical, concerning his academic ability and his behavior. Both teachers perceived Andy as a bright and capable child, but felt that he was not applying himself. He did not appear to be working up to his potential. The teachers each noted the same behavior problems, "Andy is too silly and too social."

Paul and I tried everything imaginable to motivate Andy. We earnestly praised his neat, well done papers. We devised written contracts with him, with enticing rewards for nice work. We sternly lectured him about his behavior. Nothing seemed to help for more than a few days at a time.

Finally, a friend, aware of our school dilemma, came across a magazine article that she thought might provide us with some insight, and perhaps the key to solving the problem. The article simply suggested that too much responsibility can cause young children, particularly boys around six or seven years old, to act silly or giddy.

As we pondered over this theory, we tried to decide how it applied to our own seven year old son. Eventually, the puzzle pieces started to interlock. We began to recognize how we were guilty of placing Andy under undue pressure at home. School had been his escape. It was his place to relax, socialize, giggle and act silly. School had provided him with a deserved break from work. Whereas, home required his greatest effort!

We were amazed at how easily we had fallen into this trap. In an attempt to remedy the situation, we lifted all responsibility from Andy, except caring for himself. We still expected him to make his bed, brush his teeth, and toss his dirty clothes down the chute. Paul and I temporarily refrained from asking additional favors of him. Gradually Andy buckled down at school, and began excelling in his work. By third grade, Andy was even selected to participate in the gifted/ enrichment program at his school!

While on the subject of children and school, I believe it is advantageous to make my children's teachers aware of my disability. I typically start the school year by sending a brief note after the first day, to each of the children's elementary teachers. My letter opens with thanks to the teacher for giving my child a smooth and pleasant first day of school. Then, I openly confide in them about my disability, and briefly describe some of the symptoms that they might notice throughout the school year. The letter invites them to freely ask me any questions they may have concerning the disease. The note closes by again acknowledging my gratefulness to the teacher for his or her efforts with the students.

As illustrated earlier, it is difficult to tell how others perceive me. I may feel the Parkinson's is well hidden, when in fact, people are puzzled by traits they see. I also want to promote understanding for those unplanned occasions when something goes wrong, and my symptoms are suddenly magnified. My letter clears the air to avoid misconceptions. It also provides an explanation for my disinterested stares during parent/teacher conferences, and my hesitancy at volunteering to help with certain activities.

One final comment concerning children, is that I strongly believe parents should share with their children the commitment to find a cure. Not only does this give a family a common goal to work toward, but it also encourages children to maintain their hope for the future.

I was touched when talking with Nikki Jones, a fifteen year veteran of Parkinson's, about her family's involvement in an annual walkathon to raise research money for the American Parkinson Disease Association. One year the walkathon had fallen on the same day as her sixteen-year-old daughter's church confirmation. When Nikki assured Juli that they could skip the walkathon, and instead, have a special celebration in her honor following the religious ceremony, her daughter was adamantly opposed to such an idea. Committed to both events, Juli suggested, "We don't need to miss the walkathon! We can do both! I will take my extra clothes with me. Then, after the church service, we can go to the walkathon." Juli obviously felt a strong conviction to work toward obtaining that cure.

Most young children are, by nature, optimistic and confident about what the future holds. Their faith has not yet been tainted by life's pain and sorrow. Children can believe in the unbelievable, without question or doubt. They can, thereby, be a tremendous source of strength and encouragement to others. My own children renew my hope daily when I listen to their bedtime prayers which habitually close "...and help the doctors find a cure for Parkinson's." They never cease hoping for a miracle!

One evening during dinner, Andy inspired us with a story he had learned at school that day about Harriet Tubman, the courageous black woman who led over 300 slaves to freedom via the Underground Railroad. In a nutshell, the story told how a serious head injury sustained by Harriet Tubman was later responsible for saving her life. (There were too many significant details omitted from Andy's version for me to be able to render a full account!) Regardless, the message in the story, according to Andy, was that good can arise out of bad. Andy followed up the story by sharing his own revelation, "You know, Mom, I was thinking.

97--Parkinson's

Maybe, someday, something really great will come out of your having Parkinson's disease!"

Along with a natural ability to be positive thinkers, children possess the commendable gift of being able to overlook outer appearances--the tremors, the twitches and the frozen stature, and see the real person within. They are such nonjudgemental beings. One afternoon, I was fishing for additional ideas for this chapter on the children. I posed the question to Andy, "In what ways am I different because of Parkinson's?" After pondering briefly over my inquiry, Andy replied, "Gee, Mom, you look just like every other mom to me!" Although I feel certain that, with some prompting, he could have recalled some obvious differences attributable to my disability, Andy's response reflected how unimportant outward appearances are in the eyes of a child, and how moms are ALWAYS perfect!

Becky recently confirmed that theory. After an exhausting, but fun-filled week-end of camping with our friends, Fred and Annette Fellion, we were packing our belongings to prepare for the long journey home. Becky observed from the sidelines, as Annette rolled up sleeping bags, disassembled the tent, and boxed up pots and pans. Finally, Becky scolded, "Slow down, Annette! You're going too fast!" Apparently Becky has become so accustomed to my snail's pace that she no longer views me as abnormally slow. Rather, the rest of the world is just incredibly fast!

Parkinson's disease has become a natural part of my children's everyday lives. During another camping excursion--this time at Mark Twain State Park in northeastern Missouri, Paul and I overheard Becky and Stephanie organizing themselves to play "house". Becky quickly claimed the title of "Mother", leaving Stephanie to play the role of "Father". Stephanie, being the third born and a middle child, has always been most accomodating and easy-going. She compliantly assented to Becky's terms, but bargained, "I will play the dad, but I will have the Parkinson's disease." It is nice to be loved--just the way I am!

Chapter 6
A Laughing Matter

As I touched on briefly in the previous chapter, a sense of humor can be an invaluable tool to use in coping with Parkinson's. Laughter combats fear, stress, depression, anger and embarrassment. One quote, printed in the newspaper years ago, has stuck with me: "It takes 72 muscles to frown, but only fourteen to smile."

Quite possibly, those fourteen muscles, used for smiling, do not perform the job as well as they once did for the Parkinsonian, but that does not mean the person no longer smiles. The grins are just no longer visible to the outside world.

Mary Heitman has a remarkable ability to read and interpret her husband, Bill's, thoughts and feelings. One evening, when we had invited the Heitmans over for dinner, Paul and Bill were taking turns, as they often do when they are together, amusing the group with their witty remarks. After one particularly humorous comment by Paul, Mary glanced over at Bill's virtually expressionless face, and then observed, "Bill is getting a real charge out of that one!" Mary had not missed the sparkle in his eyes, the subtle change at the corners of his mouth, and the unmistakable glow in his face, when he heard something comical.

There are many humorous discrepancies with Parkinson's disease. For instance, I have often pondered as to why it is, my hands can shake at astronomical rates of speed when I am trying to aim that flimsy, thin strand of thread through the diminutive eye of a needle. Yet, the tremor is nonexistent, and my hands are frozen in midair, when I am holding a thermometer or a bottle of salad dressing that needs to be shaken!

Or, why is it, my head can be overruled by the prevailing forces of dyskinesia, ordering it to jerk, jolt or bob incessantly, when I am sitting in the chair at the dentist's? But, when someone asks me a simple yes or no question, and I try to nod or shake my head in response, it is cemented onto my neck, refusing to budge!

Or, how come I can only move at a snail's pace when chasing our frisky and cleverly elusive puppy, as she dodges merrily through the neighborhood? Yet, I am overcome by the powers of festination, urging me to push, shove, or stampede over anyone who happens to be in my path, while I am in the slowly advancing line leading to the altar rail in church to receive communion!

Or, why is it that my voice does not carry as far as to the person sitting right beside me, even though it feels as if I am yelling at the top of my lungs? But, when I intentionally lower my voice to inform Paul of a hidden stash of candy, four little people immediately appear, begging, "Can we have some candy, too?"

Or, how come I can not show any expression on my face--not even a trace of a smile, when someone has just shared a hilarious joke with me? Yet, when Becky proudly presents Gina, modeling the new hairdo which

Becky has created for her, with three dozen barrettes forming three dozen little antennae coming out of her head, and I am asked, "Well, what do you think, Mom?", try as I may, I can't keep a straight face to hold back the laughter long enough to reply, "Lovely!"

Or, where is the thrill in receiving a beautifully wrapped present, complete with brightly colored wrapping paper, covered with sticky tape, and sturdy ribbons circling the package and tied up in stubborn knots? Add to this, a box inside, stapled securely shut, harboring layers upon layers of tissue paper enclosing the surprise gift. What is the difference between that, and jailing the gift with lock and key, and tossing out the key?! And to think the giver could have saved on time and money, but still provided the challenge, by merely placing the gift in a brown paper bag and rolling the ends closed!

Or, why do I continue to use the expressions, "in a minute" or "just a second," when I really mean "in an hour" or "just half an hour?" And, why does Paul still bother to tell me to "hurry up," "hold still," or "take your time?"

Or, why isn't every neurologist suffering from paranoia, or an inferiority complex? Their long days are spent talking with numerous Parkinson's patients who never smile, laugh, nod, relax, or look the least bit attentive or interested in the conversation!

I have also contemplated, strictly out of curiosity, how many people I have conversed with over the past few years, who, unaware of my tendency to speak in a quiet, subdued voice, have erroneously concluded that they were losing their hearing, and have promptly scheduled an appointment with a hearing specialist!

The ability to laugh at the Parkinson's, and hence, at myself, not only relieves a great deal of stress, but also communicates an important message to other people. Lighthearted banter clearly conveys my attitude of acceptance toward the disease, and dismisses the need for others to feel sorry for me. It also invites them to see the humor in my illness, as well. Because laughter supersedes awkward tension and uneasiness, the door is open for people's questions, and dialogue, in general, pertaining to Parkinson's.

My approval of jests, aimed at my disability, has obviously been imparted to our family. One evening, Paul and I were enjoying a game of cards with my in-laws. In keeping with my conviction that I should do as much as possible for myself, I was sharing the responsibility of shuffling and dealing the cards. It did not take very many rounds, with me as the designated dealer, before the others were conditioned to seize the opportunity to use the bathroom or to refill their drinks. Shuffling and dealing are tedious and painstaking skills for me, and not something that can be rushed.

Following one hand of cards, it was once again my chore to shuffle and deal. Paul's mother hopped up from her chair, and politely asked, "Do I have time to use the bathroom?" My father-in-law glanced quickly around the table to see whose turn it was to be the dealer, and then replied with a fiendish grin, "Hell, you have time to take a bath, and even wash your hair, if you want!"

103--Parkinson's

Paul and I are die-hard card players! I am a natural for playing cards, with my inherent poker face! During another evening of socializing and card playing, we were at Paul's brother and sister-in-law's home. Paul's brother, David, had sliced open his finger that day, on the honed blade of an exacto knife. That night, as we played "Pitch", David was encumbered by the massive layers of bandage wrapped around his injured finger. After losing one round of Pitch, Marie teasingly pointed out her husband's error that had led to their defeat. David stared pathetically at his bandaged wound, and attempted to excuse his blunder by groaning, "Give me a break. I have a handicap." I came back with a snappy retort, "Yes, but so do I!"

I have earned the deserved reputation around our house as the chief procrastinator when it comes to mending projects. The simple task of sewing on a button, is a horrendous ordeal for me. The entire procedure, which takes the average person three to five minutes, can easily be prolonged into a 20 to 25 minute chore, depending on how nimble, steady and cooperative my fingers are at the given time. One morning, as Paul and I were getting dressed, a button popped off the cuff of my blouse sleeve. With an agitated sigh, I uttered, "Well, I guess it's time to throw this blouse away!"

At one of our monthly support group meetings, one young man was describing the side effects he was incurring as a result of his medications. He had been experiencing terrible nausea, often forcing him to vomit. He was also being tormented by an almost unbeatable urge to fall asleep throughout the day. After hearing his complaints, someone from the group advised, "It sounds to me like you're pregnant!"

Another support group friend, Norm Mackie, battles constantly with paralyzing bouts of rigidity. One afternoon, Norm was visiting at our home when he experienced one such attack. With his feet bolted firmly to the floor and his arms frozen to his sides, Norm looked most uncomfortable, conformed to the chair, but he continued to chatter away. When I remarked at how unaffected his speech was by the Parkinson's, Norm's face lit up, and there was the vestige of a smirk. He then explained, "I have to keep on talking or else I'm liable to be covered with a coat!"

Paul and I had the good fortune of attending the biannual conference of the American Parkinson Disease Association in New Orleans during the summer of 1990. It was extremely informative, as well as uplifting, to meet people from all across the country, who either personally fought Parkinson's, or else, worked closely in some aspect with the Parkinson's community. Included were chapter presidents, support group leaders, information and referral center coordinators, and spouses of Parkinsonians.

At the welcoming reception, the APDA director, Frank Williams, opened his speech with a bit of humor, "For a moment this afternoon, I thought New Orleans was having an earthquake. The hotel was really moving and shaking. Then I realized, it was just all the conference guests arriving!"

105--Parkinson's

Since the advent of L-dopa, it is almost impossible, at times, to discern the Parkinsonians from their counterparts. It became a dubious challenge at the APDA conference to differentiate the "haves" from the "have nots." Greg and Arlette Johnson, a young couple attending the conference from California, won the prize for stumping the most people. Greg had a prosthesis in place of a leg. He had a very lopsided gait, as he dragged his rigid right leg along. Greg was also a tad slower and less steady when seating himself, or rising from a chair, since he had to do all the work for his artificial limb. Arlette, on the other hand, concealed her Parkinson's remarkably well, especially considering she had been diagnosed for four years. It became quite amusing that week, as one person after another approached Greg, and confidently inquired, "And how long have you had Parkinson's?"

Prior to our New Orleans trip, I was feeling somewhat apprehensive about participating in a panel discussion during the conference, with other leaders of young Parkinson's support groups. I was leery about speaking in front of an audience of over two hundred listeners. It was too predictable. If I were tense, I would ramble through my part at an exorbitant rate of over ten words per second, without ever enunciating the consonants in words, using inflection in my voice, or pausing to breathe. The remainder of my symptoms might also be unveiled! I dreaded the stress of such a situation.

Upon our arrival back home to St. Louis, friends and family were anxiously waiting to hear about our trip. Aware of my apprehension concerning my presentation on the panel, many were especially eager to learn how I had fared. I responded, "There were so many people down there who were shaking, twitching, jerking, shuffling, and whose speech was hard to comprehend, that I figured there was no way I was going to stand out in the room as odd--no matter what I did. Realizing this took away all the fear, and I did perfectly!"

One afternoon, I had the privilege of getting to know Jack Stack, an especially upbeat and amusing man, who has used humor to fight Parkinson's disease (or "the monster," as Jack refers to it), for eleven years. Upon meeting someone for the first time, Jack routinely discloses his disability, and then shares with them some of his many jokes about Parkinson's, in order to alleviate any awkward uncomfortableness or embarrassment. Much of his banter is intended to poke fun at his tremors. For example, his openers when we initially met one another were:

"One favorable aspect of Parkinson's is that it has simplified my legal procedures. I no longer have to get a lawyer in order to sign a contract, I just 'shake' on it!"

"I once tried to milk a cow. But by the time I was finished, the cow was giving butter!"

"My favorite drink is a 'shake'. My favorite meal is Parkinson's chicken. It is so easy to prepare. Just 'shake' and bake!"

"I always figured that if I ever lost my job, I could get a job at Sear's--replacing the machine that shakes the paint cans!"

107--Parkinson's

A sense of humor is a very effective coping mechanism with Parkinson's. It is quite difficult to feel depressed or angry at the same time you are laughing!

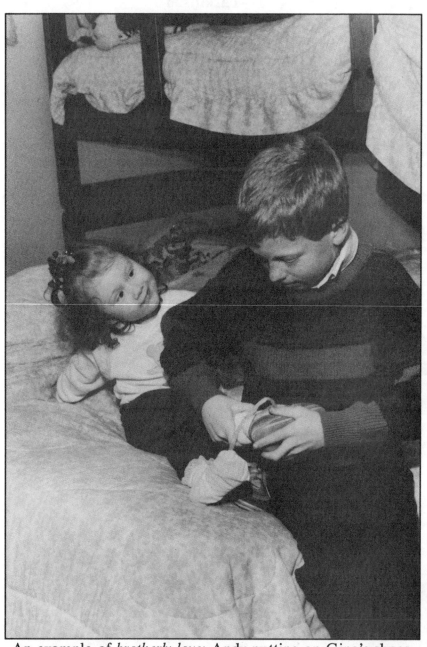

An example of *brotherly love*: Andy putting on Gina's shoes.

Chapter 7
Setting Goals

As is frequently the case when someone has been struck by misfortune, my priorities in life changed after I was diagnosed with a progressive and incurable disease. It was necessary to reassess the importance of each of my former goals, both short- and long-term goals, and to adapt them accordingly.

One of my first realizations was that I could not expect to accomplish the same number of tasks in a given day as I had before the onset of Parkinson's. Some things had to give. Even though medications may bring my speed and dexterity up to, or near par, it is very unlikely that my entire day will run smoothly. It is necessary to accommodate for my "off" periods, when my feet and hands feel as though they are weighted down, and every job requires two or three times longer to complete. What once took fifteen minutes to do, now may need thirty or more minutes to finish.

Since the length of each day can not be increased, I instead, mentally prioritize my daily goals. People come before things! My family, Paul and the children, take precedence over the dirt cowering behind the refrigerator, the cobwebs dangling from the ceiling, and the dust that collects on top of the chandelier. The chores that rank near the bottom in importance, have either been scratched completely, or else are assigned to someone else.

Ironing was one of the first jobs to be abandoned. I now refuse to purchase any clothes that need to be pressed. When Becky was visiting her grandma for a week one summer, she curiously stared at that odd, triangular-shaped thing with the steam puffing out of it that Grandma was rubbing back and forth over her clothes. Then she naively asked, "What IS that?"

I also quit carefully folding the children's clothes and stacking them neatly into their drawers, only to later discover that the drawer had been ransacked, and was in complete disarray despite my efforts. Most chores I desisted from doing, such as towel drying the pots and pans, were never missed by anyone.

Close friends and family are fantastic when it comes to doing those less urgent jobs, such as cleaning ovens and washing windows. The nicest part is, it is never necessary to ask, as they are terrific at spotting a need and volunteering their services. I have learned to never let pride interfere with accepting help by simply reminding myself that it will free my days for the more important things in life--working a jigsaw puzzle with one of my children, watching a movie alongside Paul or reading an interesting book.

In order to rid myself of any guilt at the close of the day over jobs never accomplished, Paul has cleverly advised me to ask myself such questions as, "Will the kids rot without their baths?" or "Will our guests inspect the inside of the drawers, cabinets or closets?"

Because I have learned to eliminate frivolous tasks, and to recruit the help of friends, or even hire a professional service, I have managed to conserve time and energy, which frees me for my top priorities. I have also learned the art of simplifying many tiresome, but mandatory chores. There are countless ways to simplify our daily lives, from purchasing ready-made spaghetti sauce to using automatic car washes. Even though we operate on a tight budget, sometimes my time is worth the extra expense.

One Easter, Paul and I stumbled upon a great time-saver. Determined to attend the Easter sunrise service even though the children were still very young, we came up with this creative plan. We bathed, and then, dressed each of our daughters in their fancy petticoats, frilly dresses and lacy socks the night before. On Easter morning, Paul and I crawled out of bed at 5:30 a.m., got ourselves dressed and ready. We then slipped the children's shoes onto their feet, and carried them out the door, grabbing a plastic container of Cheerios as we left. Since the advent of permanent press clothes, our children looked "no worse for the wear." The congregation was astonished by our ingenuity, and to this day, still talk about "the Easter when the Gordon family...."

Reducing my daily expectations, as well as cutting corners whenever possible, not only allows me more time for my most meaningful goals, but also cuts back considerably on stress. Trying to keep up with all my pre-Parkinson's activities is a sure fire way to invite frustration, and consequently, impair my efficiency even more. It is not possible to do it all anymore!

Another piece of wisdom, acquired from other Parkinsonians I have met, is to not postpone future dreams or goals, if at all possible. Pat Schark, a bright and extremely positive woman in our support group, wisely decided one day, that it made no sense to plan that dream vacation to Hawaii, or to schedule that trip white water rafting on the Rio Grande and hiking through the Grand Canyon, after the children were all married, college educated, or off on their own. Realizing that Parkinson's disease follows no set pattern, and progresses at a most unpredictable pace, Pat resolved to enjoy these trips now, when she could foretell the extent of her symptoms. Pat and her husband began lining up their vacations for several upcoming summers, and today, happily retell stories of these memorable expeditions.

Another tip pertaining to setting goals, is that it can be very rewarding to periodically challenge yourself with a more difficult ambition. One hobby I haven't yet relinquished, is baking and decorating my children's birthday cakes. Having learned the art of cake decorating B.P. (before Parkinson's), I have constructed some elaborate cakes--clowns, castles, bunnies, airplanes, racing cars, etc. Determined to hold on to this delicate skill as long as possible, I have literally spent eight hours working on some of my creations! I motivate myself when each birthday rolls around, by recalling the look of delight and pride in my children's eyes, as they excitedly inform each guest, "My mom made this cake!"

From time to time, I get nonsensical yearnings to try some skill that had been previously renounced because of my disability. Having fought off these desires at one time, because of practicality, I now realize the great therapeutic value in pursuing SOME of these challenges. It can be so revitalizing to prove to myself that I am still capable of performing certain skills, even though it may take twice as long.

For instance, one summer I had an unrelenting urge to sew again. I probably made four or five trips to the store and browsed through pattern books, only to end up talking myself out of this crazy idea, and leaving empty-handed. At $5 or more for a pattern, plus the soaring cost of material and notions (not to mention time!), I knew I could purchase practically any article of clothing at the discount stores for less than it would cost to sew it. And, I reasoned that I had neither the time, nor the steady hand, to do all that pinning, cutting, threading, and stitching. It had been approximately five years since I had sewn anything. Yet, I could not combat this persistent craving to sew.

Finally, one afternoon I caught myself strolling out of the fabric store, with a bag of goodies in my hand. I had done it! There was no turning back now! Much to my amazement, my symptoms were minimal whenever I sat down at the sewing machine to work on my projects. This could likely be attributed to the fact that I was doing something I really wanted to do.

About four weeks later, I proudly showed off Becky's two jumpers, and my two skirts and a blouse to anyone who innocently asked what I had been up to lately. The sense of accomplishment at that moment was well worth the late nights, and the occasional aggravation. Plus, I had satisfied and put to rest, my unremitting urge to sew--at least for another five years!

Attempting a skill totally out of the realm of my capabilities would not, of course, foster a sense of pride. Rather, this would only create unneeded frustration. My neurologist, Dr. Tempel, has also cautioned me against ever succumbing to a penchant that could result in physical harm. He gave me this warning after I proudly recounted a week-end camping trip, during which I had tried and succeeded at water skiing, for the first time in ten years. Although I did not feel I took any undue risk, Dr. Tempel's point is well taken.

Sometimes my urges have challenged me to master a brand new skill. For example, recently I longed to learn to play the guitar. Fully aware that this feat would not be easy, and perhaps not even possible, I undertook this calling with the attitude, "nothing ventured, nothing gained." Deciding I could chalk it up to experience if the skill was beyond my capabilities, I obtained an inexpensive, used guitar from a friend, who is a notorious garage sale shopper. I purchased a "teach yourself" music book, and set to work. I can not give you the outcome of this venture, as I am still trying to get past the first lesson! However, I can attest that my vibrato is wonderful!

As was the case when I sat down to sew for the first time in five years, Parkinson's symptoms are often minimal when I am doing something that I fervently wish to do. A great illustration of this phenomenon involves our good friend, Bill Heitman. Rarely have we spent an evening with Bill when he has not had to contend with either a distracting bout of dyskinesia, or a confining state of rigidity.

One rainy spring day, Paul and Bill had planned to attend an open house at a local air force base. The foul weather did not alter their plans. Bill is a former weapons system officer/navigator of fighter planes and light bombers, and has a passionate interest in airplanes. He and Paul braved the weather, wandering amid the various planes on display, and watching the shortened air show during a break in the rain. Throughout the six or seven hours they spent together, Paul attested that Bill did not once appear dyskinetic or symptomatic. Bill had done remarkably well, because he was in a familiar environment doing exactly what he loved!

I also advocate that Parkinsonians include in their lives, activities in which they can be of service to others. Parkinson's can be such a disabling disease that its victims all too often find themselves locked in the role of the dependent. It becomes tiresome, and mentally unhealthy to always be the one in need, and on the receiving end. It is such a psychological boost to be able to reach out and help others, and to do the giving for a change.

Soon after Gina's birth, a dear church friend, Yvonne Baker, offered to have Becky and Stephanie over one afternoon each week to play with her children, providing me with a needed break and time alone with the baby. As if that wasn't enough, Yvonne always brought dinner (complete with a dessert!) when she returned the girls. This routine went on for about two months.

Two years later, Yvonne gave birth to her third child. In a feeble attempt to repay her kindness, I volunteered to bring her family dinner one evening, remembering how difficult it was to prepare a meal with a newborn in the house. Yvonne graciously accepted my offer. I have a feeling Yvonne knew as well as I that, even though she was recuperating from the Caesarean delivery of her new son, it was probably less taxing for her to cook their dinner than for me. However, Yvonne was insightful enough to know that I wanted and needed to do this favor, and so never put up an argument. I will always appreciate this. There is no greater feeling than that which you get from giving of yourself, in whatever capacity you are capable of, to help others.

Another piece of advice, learned from fellow Parkinsonians, is to build safeguards into your career, JUST IN CASE. Having an alternate career plan is good common sense if you are not financially or mentally prepared to retire early. This is particularly important for surgeons, pilots, truck drivers, and other occupations that require precise skills which may, eventually, become too difficult for a Parkinson's sufferer.

One young man in our support group had a private dental practice at the time of his diagnosis. He immediately explored the possibility of teaching dentistry at a local university. He wisely sought a career option in the event that he could no longer maintain his practice.

It is of utmost importance that all Parkinsonians set a goal that commits them to some form of daily exercise. Staying physically fit is an aspiration everyone should adopt, but especially a person combating Parkinson's. It is vital because of their natural tendency toward immobility. An exercise program can positively affect balance, coordination, and mobility, and thus, encourage continued independence in the various activities of daily living. I adhere to the slogan, "Use it, or lose it!" Once a skill is surrendered, it becomes very difficult to later regain. The underlying rule is, the more a person with Parkinson's does for himself, the better off he will be in the long run.

A good starting place for deciding the most suitable type of exercise regime, would be to schedule a visit with a physical therapist. A competent physical therapist is trained to evaluate a patient's needs, and to prescribe an individualized program to serve those needs. Stretching exercises, which enhance and preserve a range of motion in all of the major joints, (shoulders, elbows, wrists, ankles, knees and hips), are more essential than exercises geared at building strength. Engaging in a strenuous or inappropriate exercise program could even be very harmful.

However, with a doctor or physical therapist's approval, a person with Parkinson's can continue virtually any form of exercise with which they were involved at the onset of the illness. The types of exercise routines, used by the various members of our support group, range from work-outs at local physical fitness centers, to simple calisthenics or a daily walk.

In addition, most members also perform some range of motion exercises, outlined by a physical therapist, or following along with a video cassette tape, specifically designed for Parkinsonians.

Upon receiving my diagnosis of Parkinson's and realizing the value of staying in shape, I sampled numerous methods of obtaining exercise, including riding a stationary bike, jogging in place, and using an exercise album. Finally, I stumbled on the key factor for deciding the best form of exercise for myself. It was mandatory that the activity selected, be one which I sincerely enjoyed. Otherwise, I inevitably failed to remain motivated, and once my enthusiasm fizzled out, so did my exercising.

For me, the most gratifying form of exercise is a daily two to five mile walk. I am most apt to remain faithful if I can incorporate the walk into my day, so that it will be accomplishing two or more things at once, rather than making the walk strictly exercise. Since Becky needs to be escorted to and from school daily, we have abandoned the van, and have resolved to make the two mile round trip on foot. I get my needed exercise, Becky gets to school and back safely, and Gina and Stephanie get an outing and some fresh air. One further bonus is the walks provide an opportune time to converse with the girls without interruption. Becky is much more likely to share the news of her day on our strolls, without the distractions at home of neighborhood playmates, television, or toys.

Another motor activity, which also operates under the principle of "Use it, or lose it," and which also may require specific daily exercise, is speech. It is estimated that about one half of all Parkinson's sufferers encounter speech difficulties, which may include a decrease in volume, changes in the quality of the voice, an increase in the rate of speaking, or poor articulation. [4] I happen to be one of the more unfortunate souls, who possess essentially every one of the possible symptoms related to speech.

It is my own personal belief that virtually every Parkinson's sufferer experiences some change, however subtle, in their speech. These symptoms are often the last to be noticed, or at least, admitted to, by the patient. I have conversed with numerous Parkinsonians who have stated unequivocally that their speech hasn't been affected in any way by the Parkinson's. Yet, as they were speaking, these same people stuttered, slurred words or spoke in a monotone or soft voice. It is especially difficult to realize when your volume of speech has diminished.

A certified speech-language pathologist can best assess a person's problems, and recommend a treatment program to help manage the difficulties. The American Parkinson Disease Association has published an excellent booklet, entitled "Speech Problems and Swallowing Problems in Parkinson's Disease".[5] I try to follow their speech improvement exercises each day, and have experienced a dramatic effect on my speaking.

The exercises are to be completed, ideally, in front of a mirror. Mirrors provide visual feedback on the movements of the lips and tongue during speech. It is also important to maintain good posture while you are practicing the exercises.

The problem of speaking too quietly to be heard easily, is typically the first speech problem encountered by Parkinsonians. The loss of volume is the result of a decrease in movement and control of respiratory muscles. To compensate for this problem, people with Parkinson's need to condition themselves to pause for breath more frequently while talking. There are exercises to reinforce this change in habit.

To counteract the tendency to speak in a very monotone voice, there are various exercises aimed at teaching the person to use different levels of loudness, to stress key words in sentences, and to change intonation when conversing.

Poor enunciation is caused by a loss of strength and a decrease in the range of tongue and lip movements. Thus, by daily exercising the tongue, lips and jaw, the clarity of speech will be favorably affected. In addition, it is helpful to practice saying numerous words, overemphasizing the pronunciation of each consonant sound, and over-exaggerating the movements of the tongue, lips and jaw.

The problem of speaking too rapidly can be alleviated by practicing the exercises designed to improve articulation, and those intended to increase the volume of speech. By concentrating on precisely enunciating each word, and taking additional pauses for breath, the rate of speaking will be consequently slower.

My speech problems are, without a doubt, the most frustrating and the most perturbing of ALL the

Parkinson's symptoms I exhibit. It amazes me how something that was once so taken for granted, such as speaking, could now require such effort. Speech has become such an odious chore, especially during my "off" periods of the day, that I often opt for the easier route--silence. I am also less talkative during my "on" times. Because producing intelligible speech requires such deliberate concentration, conversing with others can be very stress-provoking. Stress heightens the dyskinesias which, in turn, causes me to feel very self-conscious. Thus, over time I have been conditioned to associate discomfort with talking, and thereby avoid it. People who did not know me well before the onset of Parkinson's, mistakenly have me pegged as "shy," or "timid," and would be shocked to see a glimpse of my previous outgoing nature.

Despite my avoidance of conversation at times, I still value and am very thankful for my ability to speak. Personally, I could accept the loss of fine motor coordination, the loss of mobility, ANYTHING!, more easily than the loss of communication skills. Therefore, I am willing to do all in my power to guard these skills.

It may also be necessary for some Parkinson's patients to make a personal commitment to eat three balanced meals a day. Approximately one-fourth of the Parkinson's population experience loss of weight as a result of their disability. A number of factors contribute to this "problem." (I personally view this as a problem even though many people do not!)

A first deterrent to eating healthy is the tremendous effort involved. A sizzling hot, thick, juicy sirloin steak tends to lose its appeal when I am simultaneously faced with all the work entailed to subdivide it into bite-size portions and then transport them to my mouth. Even if I coerce Paul to handle the mechanics of cutting the meat, there still remains the taxing jobs of chewing and swallowing. I haven't yet devised a solution that would enable me to pass off these chores and still provide my body with the necessary calories and nutrients to function. Secondly, there is the problem of diminished appetite. Anorexia and constipation are common side effects of many antiparkinson drugs. A poor appetite may also be a consequence of depression. Furthermore, some Parkinsonians have decreased taste and smell which detracts from the normal enjoyment of foods. Finally, because research suggests that high protein foods may decrease the effectiveness of the medications and exacerbate the symptoms, and high-carbohydrate foods may boost the effectiveness of the drugs and exacerbate the dyskinesias, you can't win for trying! "You are what you eat" carries special meaning for Parkinsonians!

A final point in this chapter is that every Parkinsonian ought to devise a goal, ANY goal, aimed at finding a cure or bettering the lives of those afflicted. Who, but a person living with the disease, has as much drive, dedication, and hope for personal gain from such a goal.

There are innumerable ways to make a difference in the outlook of the future for Parkinsonians. Goals could entail becoming politically active in issues affecting the disabled, such as the logistics of using fetal

tissue in research, the controversy over animal experimentation, the availability of social security benefits,
and the procurement of national health care insurance.
Goals could also be aimed at increasing public
awareness and education about Parkinson's. Perhaps
your interests lie in organizing or becoming actively
involved in a support group. You might wish to
compose an editorial, or magazine article on the
emotional or medical aspects of Parkinson's. Or maybe
you prefer to speak publicly at schools or other func-
tions. There are many possibilities.

Finally, goals could be directed at research. You
may decide to personally participate in a research
study, or to secure the funds for such programs, either
through making donations, or becoming involved in
fund-raisers. Research is vital to the medical community in attaining additional knowledge concerning symptoms, causes, medications, the physiology of the brain,
etc., which will hopefully lead to a cure one day. If I
don't do something--anything!!--to help myself, how can
I expect others to care enough to take part in my cause,
as well?!

Even though I try to set realistic goals in order to
keep my life purposeful, I have not given up my hopes
and dreams. I frequently tease with Paul, "When I get
cured and return to teaching, we will get caught up on
our bills." I also plan to learn calligraphy upon receiving my cure. I have always heard there is power in
positive thinking!

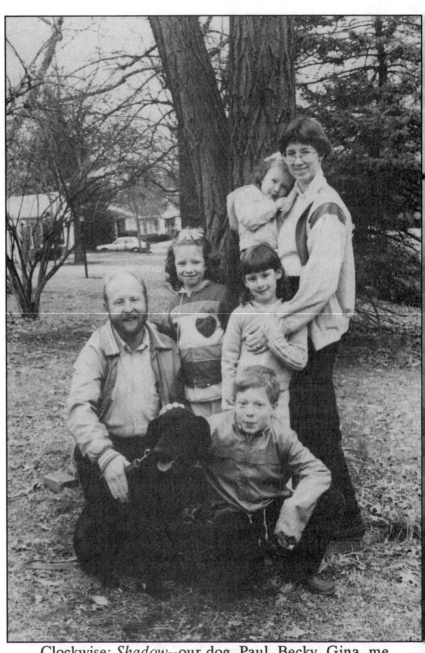

Clockwise: *Shadow*--our dog, Paul, Becky, Gina, me
Stephanie and Andy--January 1992.

Chapter 8
The "ParkinSIDEian"

The term, "ParkinSIDEian", was coined by television host and producer, Ralph Edwards, at the 1990 conference of APDA in New Orleans. In a very touching and inspiring speech, Mr. Edwards used the word, ParkinSIDEian, to refer to the counterpart of the Parkinsonian, that special person who devotedly stays at the side of the Parkinson's victim. The ParkinSIDEian may be a spouse, parent, child, friend or other significant caregiver. Mr. Edwards is a ParkinSIDEian, lovingly caring for his wife, Barbara, a long time sufferer of Parkinson's disease.

Throughout this chapter, I have used the words, "ParkinSIDEian" and "caregiver", interchangeably. For many people, "caregiver" connotes a person who assumes physical care for someone who is incapable of caring for himself. I have not chosen to confine the term, "caregiver", to this small population. The miracle of modern medicine has enabled many Parkinsonians to retain their independence, their careers, their pastimes, and quality of life for many years. However, even though physical care may be unnecessary for quite some time, other needs emerge at the precise moment that Parkinson's disease barges into someone's life. From the onset of this intruder, Parkinson's victims need someone with whom they can share their concerns or grief, someone who will show patience during those times when Sinemet is off duty, someone who will offer encouragement when frustration and defeat are rampant, someone who will love them unconditionally as their shoulders droop, their feet shuffle and their smile fades. These are examples of the kind of care provided by the "caregiver", according to my definition.

One afternoon, I was talking on the telephone with Jack Stack, a fellow Parkinsonian. He reminded me of the importance of recognizing the role of our spouses by saying, "You know, Sandi, we must not forget, as we are dealing each day with our Parkinson's, that my Betsy and your Paul have Parkinson's too." Jack was absolutely right. ParkinSIDEians' daily lives revolve totally around the disease, as well. In many respects, life is no easier for them.

It is quite natural for caregivers to traverse some or all of the stages of grief upon receiving the news that their spouse, parent, child or friend is afflicted with Parkinson's. They, too, have sustained a great loss, and may have to forfeit dreams of the future, lifestyle, relationships, personal time, and possibly, a career. Caregivers must contend with an assortment of conflicting feelings. Emotions may vacillate between anger and compassion, resentment and remorse, fear and optimism. The caregiver's days often become a string of demands which are mentally and/or physically draining.

In order to maintain a loving relationship with their disabled partner, as well as a fulfilling life of their own, ParkinSIDEians must minimize the stress in their daily lives. Many of the suggestions addressed to Parkinson's patients in the chapter on goal setting are equally applicable to the ParkinSIDEians. For starters, their daily goals must likewise be prioritized, with nonessential tasks eliminated. There is a great tendency for caregivers to be overtaxed with work and responsibility. They need to honestly admit their limitations--time, energy, and capabilities, and set reasonable and realistic goals accordingly. If they have not yet mastered the art of responding with a definitive "no" to excessive demands of their time and talents, it is imperative that they acquire this indispensable skill.

Paul can no more continue doing all that he did prior to the onset of the disease in our family, than I can. Much of what used to fall within my job description, now falls upon Paul's shoulders. He is now the one who escorts the dog to the veterinarian for her check-ups and shots. He is the one who sees to it that both vehicles are taken in for their yearly inspections, and that their licenses are purchased. In addition, there are the innumerable favors which Paul performs daily, such as buttoning that deviant button on one of my sleeve cuffs, or cutting my meat into bite-sized pieces after he has already cut up the meat for three other persons at the dinner table, not including his own!

Whereas I recommended that the Parkinsonian occasionally challenge himself with a more difficult, but highly rewarding goal to boost self-esteem, the Parkin-SIDEian also needs to pursue a hobby, a sport, a vocation, or other ambition.

Preserving an outside interest is often the key to managing the stress of caring for a disabled loved one. The chosen activity may serve as a source of enjoyment, relaxation, personal fulfillment, friendships, or income. Involvement in a favorite pastime is also beneficial in combating boredom, resentment and depression. Initially the inclusion of another commitment that demands time and energy may appear self-defeating and frivolous. However, this needed break from the work routine can ironically generate more time and energy for a caregiver. Whether it be playing a game of racquetball, refinishing an antique, teaching others the piano, activities that trigger a smile can restore vitality to caregivers, and prevent them from stagnating in life.

ParkinSIDEians, like all people, need to reserve time for themselves. Devoting their life exclusively to caring for another is not only detrimental to their well-being, but to the patient's as well. The quality of care provided will suffer if the caregiver feels trapped, overwhelmed, unfulfilled, or unhappy. Furthermore, the Parkinsonian does not profit from total dependence, physical or emotional, on one individual. Even in the case of the progressed Parkinson's sufferer who cannot manage alone, every attempt should be made to obtain backup support to relieve the caregiver.

Even though I emphatically support Paul's need for separate interests, I must confess that it is far from easy to put into practice. I still must bite my lip when it comes right down to watching Paul saunter off with his fishing pole in hand, leaving me behind with four children to entertain. It is also hard not to object when he bolts out of the house after gulping down his dinner to attend his scheduled softball game, deserting me with a sink full of dirty dishes, and with four little people to scrub, attire in pajamas, read bedtime stories to, and bunk down for the night. My job would be arduous for the average person, and I am not the "average" person by any stretch of the imagination! Yet, neither is Paul's job comparable to that of the "average" person! As toilsome as it may be to manage without him, it is still of utmost importance that Paul be encouraged to regularly escape from his responsibilities, and do something for himself. The reward comes when Paul struts through the door, his face gleaming and excitedly provides a play-by-play account of his phenomenal slide across home plate to score the tying run!

Whenever it is feasible, I also recommend that ParkinSIDEians periodically take a trip alone, even if it is just an overnight absence. Whether it be an out-of-town conference, a week-end of fishing, or a stay with family or friends, ALL people need a respite from "work," including work to which they are sincerely dedicated. No matter how much love, pleasure, or reward is involved in caring for a chronically ill person, there are bound to be some aspects, which are regarded as "work."

Furthermore, ALL people need time out from people! I firmly believe there is truth in the proverbial line, "Absence makes the heart grow fonder." Both parties profit from time apart. The Parkinsonian is reminded of the special role their caregiver plays in their life, and appreciates their services even more. The ParkinSIDEian returns rested, or at least refreshed, from their trip, more ready to face the daily challenges.

It is also imperative for caregivers to preserve valued friendships. Ironically, many people fail to keep in touch with their old friends at precisely the time when friends are most needed. Relationships are neglected because of a shortage of time and energy. Jotting a note, paying a visit, or making a phone call further deplete the waning supply. Yet, the emotional and physical support rendered by friends are worth the effort and can completely alter the ParkinSIDEian's outlook on life.

In addition to setting goals for the good of their mental health, caregivers need to attend to their physical health. Quite often ParkinSIDEians become so absorbed in caring for another's well-being that they ignore their own welfare. Mental and physical health are interrelated. A person who is physically fit is better equipped to handle the emotional demands of daily life and to maintain a hopeful prospect of the future. Thus, caregivers should participate in some type of physical exercise on a consistent basis, receive ample rest, schedule regular check-ups, and not neglect their nutrition.

Having covered the ParkinSIDEian's personal needs, I will now address their responsibilities to the Parkinsonian as a care-provider. Many needs of the Parkinson's victim are met through the joint effort of the caregiver and the care-receiver. First and foremost is the shared obligation to become well informed on Parkinson's, above and beyond the knowledge imparted by the physician at routine examinations. Treatment of Parkinson's is based primarily on theories. There are few hard, fast rules. The more resources an individual taps into, the greater the chances are of devising the optimal management plan for a Parkinson's patient. I must reiterate that support groups are an excellent place to glean life-changing ideas and information. They should not be viewed as primarily for the benefit of the Parkinsonian. Support groups are designed and intended to provide help and encouragement for BOTH the caregiver and the care-receiver. Meeting with other ParkinSIDEians who share the same frustrations, disappointments, and fears reinforces the realization that the caregiver is not alone, which can be very comforting. The meetings are not only an opportunity to receive support, but also to give support to others. Many support groups even split up into two separate groups--the Parkinsonians and the caregivers--periodically, to prompt a different kind of sharing than what occurs when everyone meets together as one group.

In addition to becoming an informed ParkinSIDEian, it is also the responsibility of the caregiver to encourage the Parkinson's patient to hold fast to their independence. Regardless of how much speedier, cleaner, neater, or easier the task at hand could be accomplished by the caregiver, they must refrain from regularly succombing to this temptation, remembering that a person battling Parkinson's must "use it or lose it!" Plus, the "simple" acts of smoothing butter evenly over a piece of bread, twisting open the stubborn lid on a jar of apple juice, and securely tying a shoelace can have a tremendous impact on the Parkinsonian's self-esteem. On the contrary, it can be very damaging to self-esteem to deny a person of his independence. Although Parkinson's victims do not benefit from being pitied or waited on hand and foot, they do benefit from reminders of their loveable characteristics. As I have stated previously, Parkinson's disease plays havoc on one's self-image. In the midst of tremors and involuntary jerks, it is tremendously uplifting for Parkinsonians to be reassured that they are loved by and still attractive to their spouse.

Likewise, Parkinson's patients need to make a special effort to profess their love to their ParkinSIDEians. Smiles, winks, warm hugs, and even words of affection do not always come readily to people with Parkinson's. Yet, how thankless the job of the ParkinSIDEian would seem if they are never shown any gratitude for their services.

Married Parkinsonians must beware. Parkinson's disease has the despicable reputation for shattering marriages. Saddled with their own separate concerns and responsibilities, spouses often neglect to reserve time and energy for their relationship with their partner. Both individuals blindly stumble through the rituals of daily living, and fail to see the inner and outer beauty which first attracted them to their spouse. By remaining alert to this tendency, and recognizing each other's emotional need to feel loved and appreciated, couples can likely ward off the potentially devastating effects of Parkinson's on their marriage.

Speaking from almost a decade of experience as a ParkinSIDEian, Mary Heitman believes it is vitally important that the caregiver bears the responsibility of planning daily outings once Parkinson's curbs the activity level of its prey. Mary advocates that even a quick trip to the store, with her husband waiting in the car, is nonetheless an opportunity to get outdoors, and is deserving of the effort. Since motivation is often lacking for a person with progressed Parkinson's to do anything except sit at home, a daily excursion counteracts a tendency toward isolation, as well as the problems incurred from being physically inactive and idle.

Leaving the security of home not only requires more physical energy and effort, but also forces the Parkinsonian to overcome at least some of the feelings of embarrassment and self-consciousness, associated with his disability. Parkinson's disease is, without a doubt, a very humbling disease. I have been stared at, whispered about, and avoided. Facing the uneducated public when I am at either end of the spectrum--very symptomatic or very dyskinetic--is probably one of the hardest things I have ever had to do. But hiding from humanity is hardly the solution. With practice, time, and determination, and prodding from the ParkinSIDEian, the Parkinson's victim should be able to cease worrying constantly about how others perceive him. Instead, he can be open to growth from new experiences, and from meeting new people. Other people are also provided an oportunity for growth from meeting him. Virtually every person possesses certain unique qualities which unknowingly touch other lives.

People thrive on social interaction. Yet, even in the company of familiar faces, this is not always an easy feat for the Parkinsonian. As mentioned earlier, I have become much more quiet and reserved due to my speech difficulties, and my concern over my symptoms and the side effects of the antiparkinson drugs. Because of my unwillingness to converse at times, I have inadvertently discouraged many friends by giving the erroneous impression that I am not interested in a closer companionship.

Another problem affecting my social life is that I have somewhat lost my identity to Parkinson's disease. Many people are so intent on being what I term a "helper friend"--running errands or offering assistance with certain tasks--that they overlook my emotional needs. I am viewed strictly in light of my illness, and no longer seen as the person I am within. Sadly, many of my closest friends have lost touch with our former relationship, and are now merely helper friends. Although this has not been the case with Paul and me, I suspect that there is a real tendency for ParkinSIDE-ians to fall into this trap, as well.

Despite the difficulties encountered, I can not overstate the importance of both the Parkinsonian and the care-provider maintaining an active social life! The best solution to the problems incurred is honesty and openness. With their heart in the right place, helper friends are likely unaware of the limitations that they have placed on the relationship. In regards to newer acquaintances, it has become necessary for me to clarify that I do not intend to appear antisocial or aloof. (Meanwhile, I am working to overcome my reticence.) One final option to satisfy the need for social contacts is to seek out companionship with other Parkinsonians and their spouses. There is no rule which dictates that fellow Parkinson's sufferers and their spouses must restrict their socializing to support group meetings!

In addition to encouraging social interaction, another task which falls within the job description of the ParkinSIDEian is to be present at neurological examinations, whenever possible. This affords both persons the opportunity to ask questions, and to hear the doctor's explanations, recommendations, or suggestions.

Many people can relate to being alone at the doctor's office, and struggling to fully concentrate on all the doctor says. However, due to the sterile atmosphere, the stress of being there, and the many questions, whirling through your mind that you must remember to ask before you leave, many of the doctor's words drift in one ear and out the other. Because this has happened to me quite frequently, I appreciate when a physician takes the time to write things down for his/her patients. This problem is also usually resolved when there is another set of ears present, absorbing the information.

Another point, in favor of Paul accompanying me to the neurologist, is that we can each offer our own perceptions as to how I am doing currently--how a change in medication has affected me, whether or not my symptoms seem to be progressing, the extent of side effects, etc. Many neurologists only see their patients for one hour every three months, or so. The appointments may be scheduled around the same time of the day, when symptoms are typically at their best or their worst. So, the doctor can not get a very complete picture from this limited examination. He must also rely on input from his patients. Since Paul and I do not always judge my status the same, we can provide the doctor with greater insight by presenting both our views.

Living with a person afflicted with Parkinson's demands flexibility on the part of the caregiver. In addition to fluctuating motor ability, many Parkinsonians experience mood swings in conjunction with their "off" periods. They may act cold and distant, and sometimes ask not to be touched. Some patients become abnormally negative when they are functioning at their worst. They may give the exact opposite response to an idea or suggestion posed during their "off" time than if it is presented perhaps twenty minutes later during their "on" time. Decision-making skills may also reflect the status of the symptoms. When the Parkinsonian is most symptomatic, the smallest obstacle inflates to a gargantuan barrior. Finally, one ParkinSI-DEian describes her husband's personality switch as resembling someone who is "possessed". He transforms into an uncharacteristically hateful and angry person on those occasions when his symptoms are exacerbated.

As for me, I display a hint of all the above during my "off" hours. I am generally more irritable, preoccupied, unambitious, indecisive and unresponsive. The ParkinSIDEian who understands and expects this split personality will fare better during those times when the least desirable traits emerge.

ParkinSIDEians play an integral part in the lives of their disabled partners, and possess certain distinguished qualities. For example, they qualify as accomplished mindreaders, able to decipher messages of laughter, frustration, sadness or joy, without the normal visual or verbal clues. Furthermore, caregivers may wear the hats of chauffeur, nurse, secretary, dietician, counselor, or physical and occupational therapist.

If that isn't challenging enough, spouses of Parkinson's sufferers must frequently relinquish an uninterrupted night's sleep if their mate is tormented by insomnia. Parkinson's disease tends to rob its victims of peaceful slumber. I have friends who typically awake numerous times each night. Unable to win the battle against insomnia, they resort to snacking, reading, or exercising to pass the time (sometimes hours!). If the ParkinSIDEian does manage to obtain eight hours of sound sleep, the pride is diminished by the guilt of knowing their mate only cat napped through the night.

Experience has taught the ParkinSIDEian to be a jack-of-all-trades. Paul has been called upon to master a broad range of skills, some of which he would not likely have acquired, if it had not been for the intrusion of Parkinson's disease. I fondly recall that shivery January morning, when Becky stood, patiently watching, as I guided her inexperienced daddy, one step at a time, through the process of braiding the thick, frizzy hair of her new Christmas Barbie doll. Eventually Paul broadened his scope and began braiding our daughters' hair!

ParkinSIDEian Charlotte Shelburne shared with our support group the story of her debut as an electrician. She and her husband, Bob, were adding a bathroom to their basement. When it came time to do the wiring in order to run electricity into the bathroom, Bob provided the know-how and Charlotte supplied the hands. Charlotte confessed that, prior to that Saturday afternoon, her knowledge of electricity went only as far as turning a light switch on and off! However, with Bob furnishing step-by-step instructions from his supervisor's post lying on a bed, Charlotte eventually accomplished the task! She has since added "plumber" to her impressive resume, as well, after replacing the sink in their upstairs bathroom!

In the eleven years that Betsy Stack has qualified as a ParkinSIDEian, she has succeeded at changing the oil in the car, doing the necessary body work on a rusty car fender, replacing a worn-out kitchen faucet, installing a garbage disposal, and refurbishing the exterior of their home with a fresh coat of paint, to name but a few of her many accomplishments. After listing all of his wife's notable attributes, Jack Stack added, "The best thing I can offer her is Inconsistency." However, just as Betsy has not limited her own capabilities, neither does she allow her husband to shortchange his abilities or to adopt a defeatist attitude. Jack believes that Betsy's high expectations for him and her unwillingness to offer sympathy are the keys to her supportive role.

Because of their abounding energy, surplus of patience, extraordinary stamina, and commendable ability to be positive thinkers, ParkinSIDEians appear to be immune to fatigue, illness or depression. (Unfortunately, this is a fallacy.) I have a tremendous respect, and the greatest appreciation, for this irreplaceable, but frequently overlooked and unrecognized, group of individuals. I propose the old adage, "Behind every successful man, there is a woman," be modified to state, "Beside every successfully coping Parkinsonian, there is a devoted, and supportive ParkinSIDEian!"

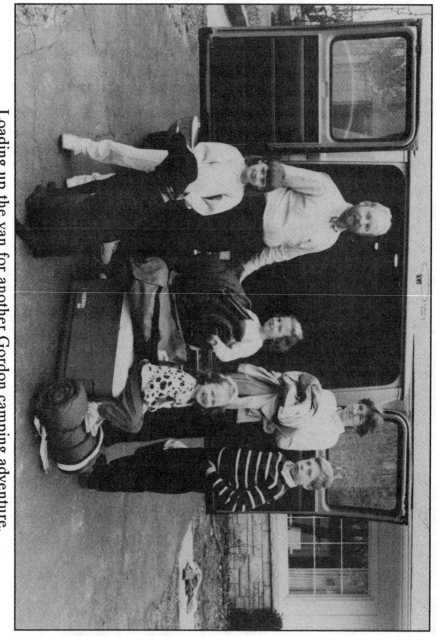

Loading up the van for another Gordon camping adventure.

CONCLUSION

In conclusion, people who respond, indefinitely, to a diagnosis of Parkinson's disease with a grim and defeated attitude, are bound to be plagued by unyielding depression, misdirected anger, painful loneliness, and lack of ambition. They are disabled to a far greater extent, than those individuals who creatively and determinedly come to an acceptance of the situation. Parkinson's disease does not have to be an indisputable sentence to a life of grief and passive constraint. No matter what physical limitations the disease poses, the afflicted are still free to smile and laugh within, bask in the warmth of friendships, and touch and affect the lives of others. They never have to surrender their hope for new treatments and their hope for a cure.

Although I would trade for another set of circumstances in a moment, Parkinson's disease has, nevertheless, opened many new doors for me. It has allowed me to appreciate all those countless motor skills, which the general population take for granted--shaking a salt or pepper shaker, rolling over in bed, reading aloud *The Cat in the Hat* to an attentive child, walking painlessly through doorways, or opening a sandwich tangled up in plastic wrap. As sad and unfortunate as it may be, people can not fully appreciate the miracles of the human body--dexterous fingers that can pick up a coin or the muscles which cooperatively work to produce speech--until they experience the frustration of living without.

I have also learned not to waste energy and time on frivolous, petty dilemmas, such as what color to paint the bathroom walls, or which outfit to wear to the party. The world is full of much greater and more worthwhile concerns. Driving safely, securely holding a baby, or even thoroughly brushing my teeth, require very deliberate care and concentration on my part.

My disability has shown the unconditional love of my devoted ParkinSIDEian, Paul, and thereby strengthened our marriage. My relationship with God has grown, too, from having a need, and witnessing God's response to that need. Parkinson's has taught our children compassion and acceptance for others, especially people who are different in some way. It has also taught them patience and independence. Parkinson's has provided me with the rich opportunity to meet dozens of inspiring and wonderful people whose paths, otherwise, would have never crossed mine.

And, my illness has created new goals and new purposes in my life.

Until the discovery of a cure, I will do my best to adopt Paul's philosophy on living. I will try not to waste precious time, brooding in sorrow, anger, or envy over the times prior to Parkinson's entry in my life. Nor will I dwell on the uncertainties of my future, futilely worrying about what direction Parkinson's will take in years ahead. Instead, I will live life in the present, being thankful every day for the marvel of each new sunrise, the delightful sound of giggling children, the warmth of hugs, the triumph of each fastened button, and the promise in every medical advancement.

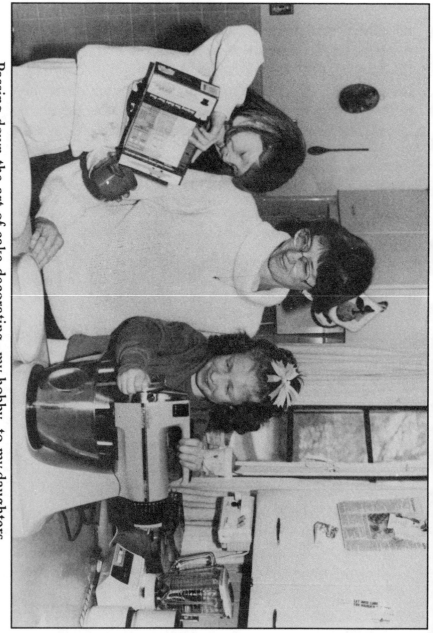

Passing down the art of cake-decorating--my hobby, to my daughters.

APPENDIX I

NATIONAL ORGANIZATIONS FOR PARKINSON'S DISEASE

The following organizations support Parkinson's research and disperse pamphlets, booklets and/or newsletters with helpful information for Parkinsonians and their families. At least one of these groups should be able to locate an information/referral center or a support group in your community.

American Parkinson Disease Association (APDA)
60 Bay Street
Staten Island, NY 10301
1-800-223-2732

American Parkinson Disease Association (APDA)
West Coast Office
13743 Victory
Van Nuys, CA 91423
818-908-9951

United Parkinson Foundation (UPF)
360 West Superior Street
Chicago, IL 60610
312-664-2344

Parkinson's Disease Foundation (PDF)
William Black Medical Research Building
650 West 168th Street
New York, NY 10032
1-800-457-6676
212-923-4700

National Parkinson Foundation, Inc.
1501 Ninth Avenue NW, Bob Hope Rd.
Miami, FL 33136
1-800-327-4545
305-547-6666

National Parkinson Foundation, Inc.
(Affiliate)
9911 West Pico Boulevard
Suite 500
Los Angeles, CA 90035
213-203-8448

National Parkinson Foundation, Inc.
(Affiliate)
122 East 42 Street
New York, NY 10017
212-867-7070

APPENDIX II
Recommended Reading Material--BOOKS:

Parkinson's Disease: A Guide for Patient and Family by
Roger C. Duvoisin, M.D. New York: Raven
Press, 1984

Parkinson's: A Patient's View by Sidney Dorros. Cabin
John, MD: Seven Locks Press, Inc., 1981

Awakenings by Oliver Sacks, M.D. New York: Harper-
Collins, 1990

From Rage to Courage: The Road to Dignity Walk by
Michel Monnot. Northfield, MN: St. Denis Press,
1988

Living Well With Parkinson's by Glenna Wotton At
wood. New York: John Wiley & Sons, Inc., 1991

Ivan: Living with Parkinson's Disease by Ivan Vaughan.
New York: MacMillan Company, 1986

When Bad Things Happen to Good People by Harold
Kushner, New York: Avon Books, 1981

The Anatomy of an Illness as Perceived by the Patient by Norman Cousins. New York: W.W. Norton and Company, 1979

We Are Not Alone: Learning to Live with Chronic Illness by Sefra Kobrin Pitzele. St. Paul, MN: Thompson & Company, Inc., 1985

Living With Parkinson's Disease: Don't Rush Me! I'm Coping As Fast As I Can by Jon Robert Pierce. Knoxville, TN: Spectrum Communications, 1989

Parkinson's Disease: The Facts by Gerald Stern, M.D. and Andrew Lees, M.D. New York: The Clarendon Press, 1982

Parkinson's Disease Handbook by Richard Godwin-Austen M.D. Baltimore, MD: International Health, 1989

Mainstay: For the Spouse of the Chronically Ill by Maggie Strong. Boston, MA: Little, Brown and Company, 1988

PAMPHLETS AND BOOKLETS:

Parkinson's Disease: One Step at a Time by J. David Grimes, M.D., Peggy A. Gray, R.N., and Kelly A. Grimes, B.Sc. Ottawa, Ontario: Parkinson Society of Ottawa-Carleton, 1989

Parkinson's Disease Handbook by A.N. Lieberman, M.D., G. Gopinathan, M.D., A. Neophytides, M.D., and M. Goldstein, Ph.D. Staten Island, NY: The American Parkinson Disease Association

Coping With Parkinson's Disease by Susan B. Levin and Erwin B. Montgomery, Jr., M.D. Staten Island, NY: The American Parkinson Disease Association, 1986

Speech Problems and Swallowing Problems in Parkinson's Disease Staten Island, NY: The American Parkinson Disease Association

Be Active! by Rose Wichmann, R.P.T., The Institute for Rehabilitation Services, Methodist Hospital, Minneapolis. Staten Island, NY: The American Parkinson Disease Association, 1990.

The Parkinson's Challenge by Jan Peter Stern, Staten Island, NY: The American Parkinson Disease Association, 1987.

Equipment and Suggestions by Marilyn B. Robinson, B.N. Occupational Therapy Department, The Burke Rehabilitation Center, White Plains, NY. Staten Island, NY: The American Parkinson Disease Association, 1989.

APPENDIX III
Exercise and Speech Video Tapes

Rhythms and Moves sold by Physical Therapy Consul
tants, 2912 Elliott St. N.W., Washington, D.C.
20008

Get Up and Go sold by Health Tapes, P.O. Box 47190,
Oak Park, MI 48237, (313) 662-5100

Keep Movin sold by Parkinson's Disease Clinic at
Methodist Hospital, P.O. Box 650, Minneapolis,
MN 55440

Speech Therapy: Parkinson's Disease sold by Lee Silver
man Center for Parkinson's, 7300 East Fourth
Street, Suite #102, Scottsdale, AZ 85251

APPENDIX IV
Government Help

This is but a sampling of the help available for Parkinson's victims. Persons in need of assistance should contact a local Medicare office, welfare office and/or Social Security office to learn their options.

MEDICARE:

Medicare is a health insurance program designed primarily for people over the age of 65 who qualify for Social Security benefits. Medicare provides hospital insurance at no cost. For a monthly premium, Medicare also offers an optional medical insurance plan which would cover doctors' services and numerous other medical services. A disabled person who is receiving Social Security Disability Insurance can qualify for Medicare after their 24th SSDI check, regardless of age.

MEDICAID:

People of any age whose income is below an allotted amount may receive assistance with doctor and hospital bills through Medicaid. This program is administered by the state, following certain federal guidelines.

People who are receiving Supplemental Security Income checks are usually able to qualify for Medicaid.

SOCIAL SECURITY DISABILITY INSURANCE:

SSDI is intended for people who are eligible for Social Security benefits, but are under 65 years of age and have become completely disabled, leaving them unable to work for at least twelve months. These funds are available five months after the disability occurs. SSDI continues for life unless the individual resumes his job, in which case the benefits are terminated after a 3-month grace period.

SUPPLEMENTAL SECURITY INCOME:

To qualify for SSI, a person must either be over 65, or blind or completely disabled, and have financial need. Total income (wages, pensions and Social Security) and certain assets (real estate, bank accounts, cash, stocks, bonds) are evaluated to determine eligibility of applicants.

VETERAN'S ADMINISTRATION ASSISTANCE:

The V.A. offers care for eligible disabled veterans.

APPENDIX V

DRUGS USED IN TREATMENT OF PARKINSON'S DISEASE

LEVODOPA:

Levodopa, or "l-dopa", is the most potent antiparkinson drug, because it changes directly into dopamine, the lacking chemical which governs movement. If this change starts outside of the brain, the levodopa loses much of its effectiveness, since dopamine cannot cross into the brain where it is needed. For this reason, levodopa is rarely administered alone nowadays, but rather in combination with an inhibitor, such as carbidopa, which prevents the conversion from occurring prior to l-dopa's entrance into the brain. Plus, straight levodopa caused many patients to experience nausea and vomiting. Dyskinesias, dizziness and mental changes are other side effects incurred.

SINEMET:

Sinemet is levodopa combined with carbidopa in a fixed ratio of 1 mg of carbidopa to 4 mg or 10 mg of levodopa (Sinemet 10/100, 25/100, 25/250). Sinemet is the most popular drug used in the treatment of Parkinson's disease today. Because carbidopa averts the wasteful conversion of levodopa to dopamine outside of the brain, Sinemet allows patients to take smaller total dosages of levodopa to receive the benefits. Besides increasing the effectiveness of the l-dopa, the addition of carbidopa reduces or eliminates the annoying side effects of vomiting and nausea, which are caused by levodopa converting to dopamine outside of the brain. Side effects still include dyskinesias, dizziness, mental changes, as well as nausea for some people.

DOPAMINE AGONISTS:
This class of drugs does not actually produce dopamine, but can create similar, although somewhat weaker, results by stimulating the dopamine receptors directly. Dopamine agonists may cause nausea, dizziness, low blood pressure, mental changes and dyskinesias. Two dopamine agonists frequently used to treat Parkinson's disease are:
  * bromocriptine (Parlodel)
  * pergolide (Permax)

DEPRENYL (ELDEPRYL):
Deprenyl is a fairly new drug given to Parkinson's patients. Deprenyl inhibits one of the enzymes, mono-amine oxidase B, that is normally responsible for breaking down dopamine in the brain. Physicians sometimes prescribe deprenyl for more advanced Parkinson's patients who are taking Sinemet but experiencing "wearing off". Deprenyl is used in this case to prolong the effect of a dosage of Sinemet. Other times, physicians prescribe deprenyl for newly diagnosed patients. This recent usage of deprenyl resulted from some evidence that deprenyl may slow progression of Parkinson's disease in people who are in

the early stages of the disease and who do not yet require treatment. This thinking is based on the fact that when monoamine oxidase B breaks down dopamine and other naturally occurring chemicals, by-products are produced that may further damage surrounding dopamine-producing cells. Thus, inhibiting this enzyme early on may actually slow the course of Parkinson's. Deprenyl has few side effects when used by itself. It may cause restlessness or, occasionally, drowsiness. However, when it is used in conjunction with Sinemet, deprenyl accentuates the side effects as well as the benefits of the Sinemet.

AMANTADINE (SYMMETREL):
Amantadine releases dopamine from the brain cells, and is thereby effective at relieving mild Parkinson's symptoms for many patients. Possible side effects include the appearance of spots or streaks on the skin, swelling of feet, and, more rarely, hallucinations or confusion.

ANTICHOLINERGICS:
Prior to the advent of levodopa, anticholinergics were the mainstay of Parkinson's treatment. Because the loss of dopamine cells causes an imbalance with another neurotransmitter, called acetylcholine, in the brain of the Parkinsonian, anticholinergics provide benefit by hindering the work of the acetylcholine and reinstating some of the normal balance. This group of drugs helps alleviate tremor and rigidity. The most common side effects are dry mouth, blurred vision, constipation and

mental changes. Some commonly used anticholinergics are:
* Artane
* Parsidol
* Cogentin
* Benadryl
* Akineton
* Kemadrin
* Pagitane

NOTES

1. Sidney Dorros, *Parkinson's: A Patient's View* (Cabin John, MD: Seven Locks Press, 1985)

2. Elisabeth Kubler-Ross, *On Death and Dying*, (New York: Macmillan Publishing, Co., Inc., 1969)

3. A.N. Lieberman, M.D. and others, *Parkinson's Disease Handbook*, (Staten Island, NY: The American Parkinson Disease Association), p. 1.

4. *Speech Problems and Swallowing Problems in Parkinson's Disease*, The American Parkinson Disease Association, Staten Island, NY.

5. Ibid

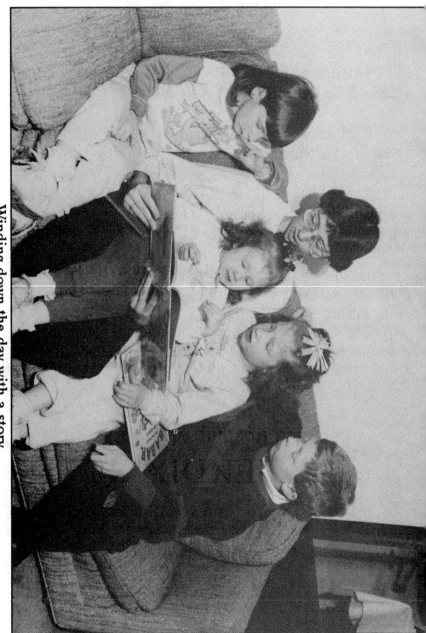

Winding down the day with a story.

INDEX

Acceptance 63, 69, 73, 76, 102
Acetylcholine 55, 155
Agility 57
Agonist 50, 154
Alert 54
Amantadine 155
Ambition 112, 127
American Parkinson
  Disease Association
  84, 95, 104, 119, 145
Amino acids 59, 60
Amitriptyline 55
Anger 46, 63, 64, 66
  83, 85, 99
Anticholinergics 55
  155-156
Antidepressant 55
Antiparkinson 56, 60, 122,
  153
Appetite 54, 122
Baker, Yvonne 115
Balance, loss of 20, 38
Ballard, Curt 77
Bargaining 63, 67
Body language 44, 79
Bradykinesia 21
Bromocriptine 154
C-section 53
Caesarean 42, 116
Carbidopa 59, 153-4
Carbohydrates 60
Career 116
Caregiver 125
Children--anger 82
Clinic 52

Compliancy 46
Compliant 45
Crying 54
Death 54
Denial 63, 64, 73
Deprenyl 154, 155
Depression 38, 53-55, 63,
  67-8, 85, 99, 122, 128
Diagnosis 37, 38, 64
  68, 73
Diet 60
Dopamine 38, 49-50, 55
  153-55
Dorros, Sidney 52
Dyskinesias 51-2, 55, 57-8
  60, 81, 83, 121-2, 153, 154
Dyskinetic 89, 133
Edwards, Ralph 125
Emotion 46, 57
Energy 54
Exercise 117, 118, 150
Expression 44, 79
Fellion, Annette & Fred
  97
Festination 22
Fright 23
Ganglia (Basal) 38
Ghost 57-8
Grief 63, 85, 126
Handwriting 20
Hastings 37, 38, 41, 49
Heitman, B & M 88
  99, 114, 133
High-carbohydrate 122
Holland, John 75

Honeymoon 50
Humor, sense 88, 99, 107
Hypersomnia 54
Independence 131
Insomnia 54, 137
Johnson, A. Greg 105
Jones, Nikki 95
Kirschbaum, Renee 71
Kubler-Ross, E. 63, 67
L-dopa 105, 153
Language 44, 79
Levin, Susan 71
Levodopa 50, 59, 60, 153
Mackie, Norm 104
Marriage 132
Medicaid 151
Medicare 151
Monet 37
Monoamine oxidasa 8
    154-5
Mood 55, 136
MRI (Magnetic Resonance
    Imaging) 38, 46, 47
National Parkinson
    Foundation 146
Nausea 41, 59, 153-4
Nerve conduction study
    17, 18
Neurotransmitter 55, 155
Newsletter 71
Parenting 80-1
ParkinSIDEian 125-6, 133
Parkinson's: A Patient's
    View 52, 147
Parkinson's Disease
    Foundation 146
Parlodel 49, 55, 154
Pergolide 154
Posture 20, 38, 44
Protein 60, 122
Rebound 53
Sadness 54
St. Louis Parkinson

Newsletter 71
Schark, Pat 112
Self-Esteem 132
Shelburne 138
Simms 35
Sinemet 39, 41, 49, 55, 59
    60, 125, 153-155
Social 134
Speech 21, 38, 119, 150
    120, 134
Spontaneity 56
SSDI 152
Stack 106, 126, 138
Starne 16-19, 27
    30, 31
Stress 23, 41, 44, 50, 57
    74, 82, 99, 126, 127
Substantia nigra 38
Suicide 54
Supplemental Security
    Income 152
Support groups 69-70
    71-73, 131
Symptom of Parkinson's
    20-1, 38
Tempel, Lee 11, 52-3
    55-56, 114
Tremor 14-18, 20, 38, 50
Tremors 38, 45, 63
Tricyclic 55
Tubman, Harriet 96
United Parkinson
    Foundation 145
Veteran's
    Administration 152
Vomiting 153-4
Walk-A-Thon 84, 95-6
Washington U. Medical
    School 52
Williams, Frank 104
Worthlessness 54